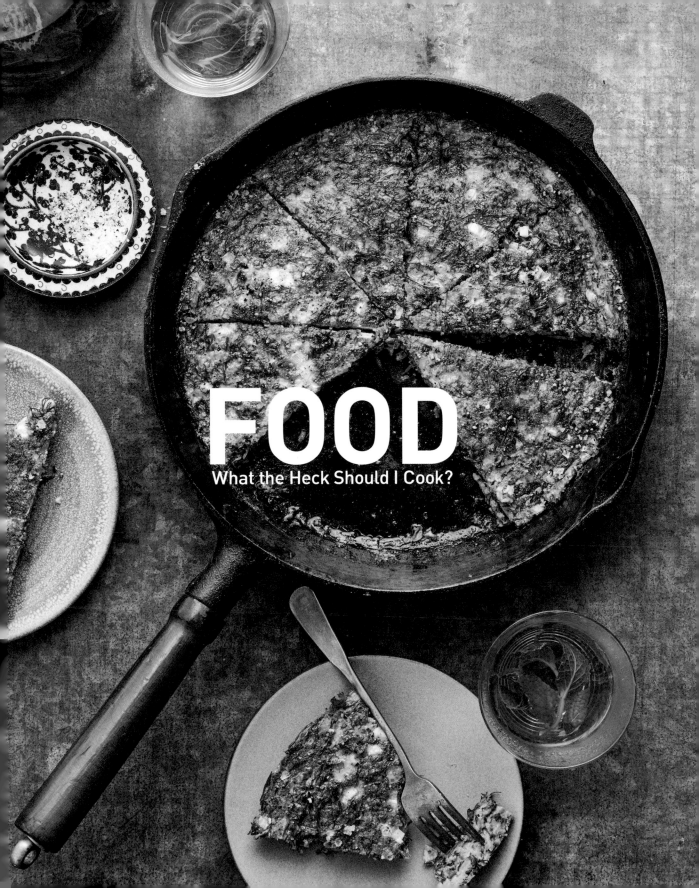

FOOD

What the Heck Should I Cook?

Books by Mark Hyman, MD

Food: What the Heck Should I Cook?

Food: What the Heck Should I Eat?

Eat Fat, Get Thin

The Eat Fat, Get Thin Cookbook

The Blood Sugar Solution 10-Day Detox Diet

The Blood Sugar Solution 10-Day Detox Diet Cookbook

The Blood Sugar Solution

The Blood Sugar Solution Cookbook

The Daniel Plan

The Daniel Plan Cookbook

UltraPrevention

UltraMetabolism

The UltraMetabolism Cookbook

The Five Forces of Wellness (CD)

The UltraThyroid Solution

The UltraSimple Diet

The UltraMind Solution

Six Weeks to an UltraMind (CD)

UltraCalm (CD)

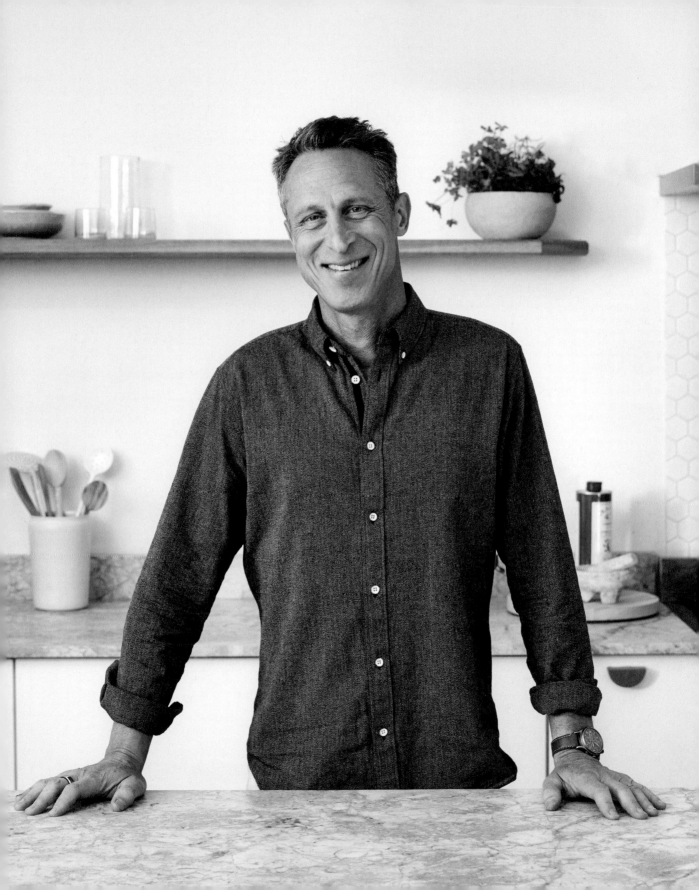

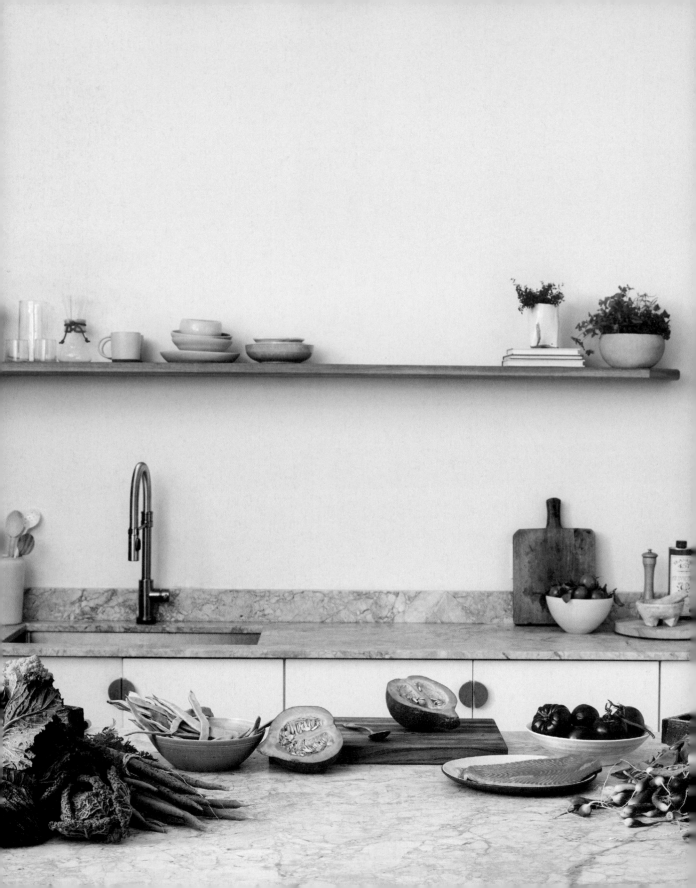

FOOD

What the Heck Should I Cook?

Mark Hyman, MD

Little, Brown Spark
New York Boston London

Little, Brown Spark
Hachette Book Group
1290 Avenue of the Americas, New York, NY 10104
littlebrownspark.com

First Edition: October 2019

Little Brown Spark is an imprint of Little, Brown and Company, a division of Hachette Book Group, Inc. The Little, Brown Spark name and logo are trademarks of Hachette Book Group, Inc.

The publisher is not responsible for websites (or their content) that are not owned by the publisher.

The Hachette Speakers Bureau provides a wide range of authors for speaking events. To find out more, go to hachettespeakersbureau.com or call (866) 376-6591.

Cover and interior design by Gary Tooth / Empire Design Studio
Photography by Nicole Franzen
Food styling by Vivian Lui
Photography props by Joni Noe

ISBN 978-0-316-45313-4
LCCN 2019937628

10 9 8 7 6 5 4 3 2 1

WOR

Printed in the United States of America

Cooking is a revolutionary act that can save our health, our economy, our climate, and our communities. To those who have never cooked, who want to cook and don't know how, or who love to cook but want to learn how to create more delicious meals to nourish body and soul, this book is for you.

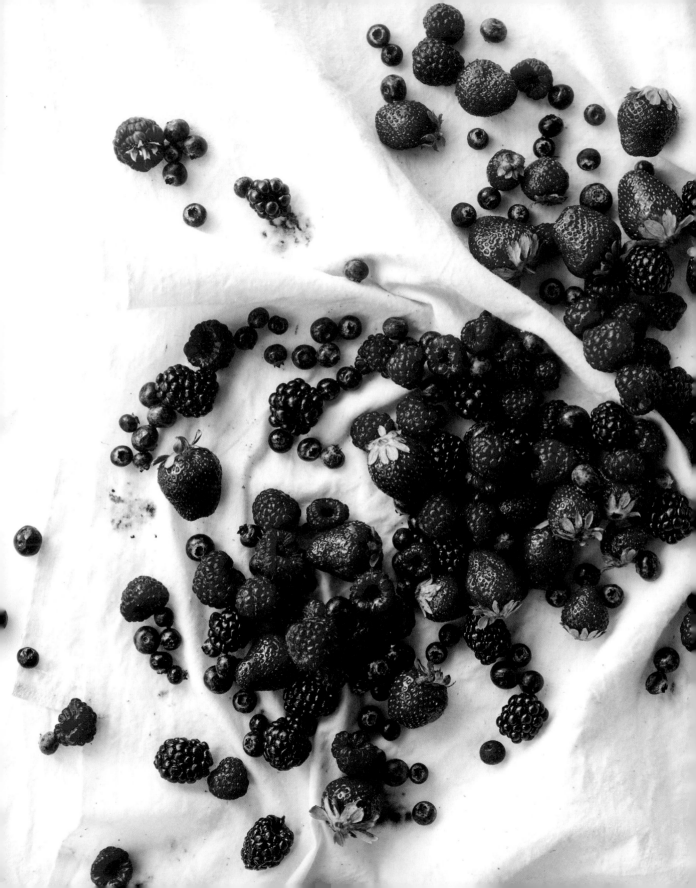

CONTENTS

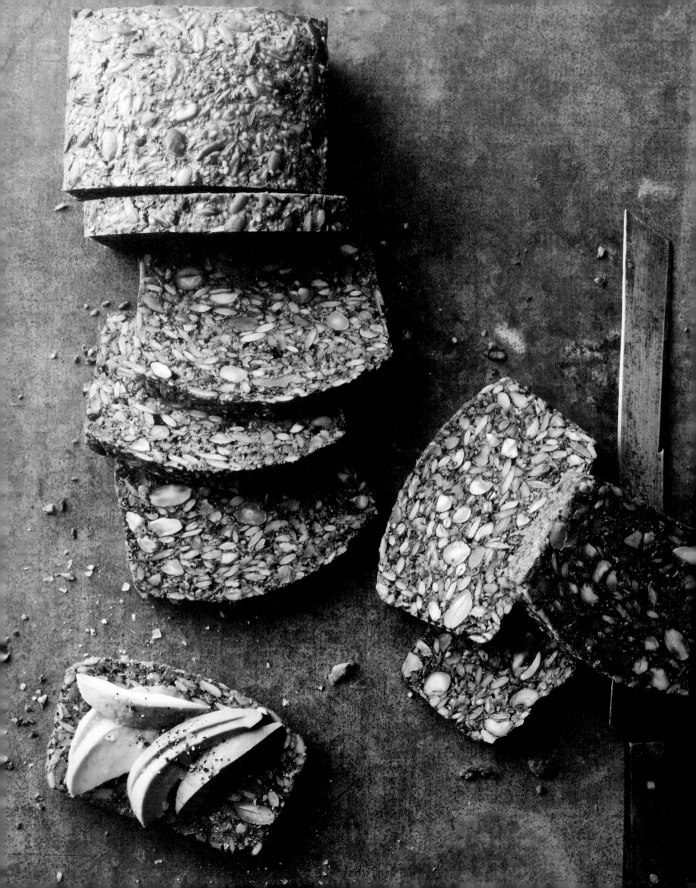

FOOD

What the Heck Should I Cook?

HOW TO USE THIS BOOK

Icons

Throughout this book, you'll see helpful icons that identify important aspects of each recipe. Everything in this book follows my Pegan Diet guidelines, so all recipes are made of real food ingredients and are gluten-free, low-glycemic, and free from unhealthy fats. Most recipes are also grain-free and dairy-free, but not all of them, and many are vegan as well. Look for the following icons to identify certain ingredients right off the bat:

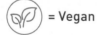 = Vegan   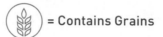 = Contains Grains   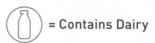 = Contains Dairy

A Little Help from My Friends

You'll notice recipes contributed by my good friends and colleagues who have realized the amazing impacts of the Pegan Diet in their own lives. I love sharing recipe ideas from others because sometimes one unique ingredient, or even a familiar one used in a creative way, can be the doorway to a new favorite meal. My recipe contributors include:

Chef José Andrés

Dave Asprey

Dr. Rupy Aujla

Mark Bittman

Chef David Bouley

Gisele Bündchen and Tom Brady

Chef Marco Canora

Kris Carr

Hugh Jackman

Dr. Deanna Minich

Dr. Mehmet Oz

Gwyneth Paltrow

Dr. David Perlmutter
  and Leize Perlmutter

Dr. Drew Ramsey

Cam Sims

Mark Sisson

Dr. Terry Wahls

Danielle Walker

I'm so grateful to these wonderful folks for joining me in sharing the goodness of real food.

I hope you are beginning to think more about your own food philosophy, identifying your personal beliefs and goals, and seeing where there is room for improvement when it comes to your dietary choices. As you read on, you'll learn much more about food quality, labeling, smart shopping, and healthful food prep to revamp your kitchen and your health.

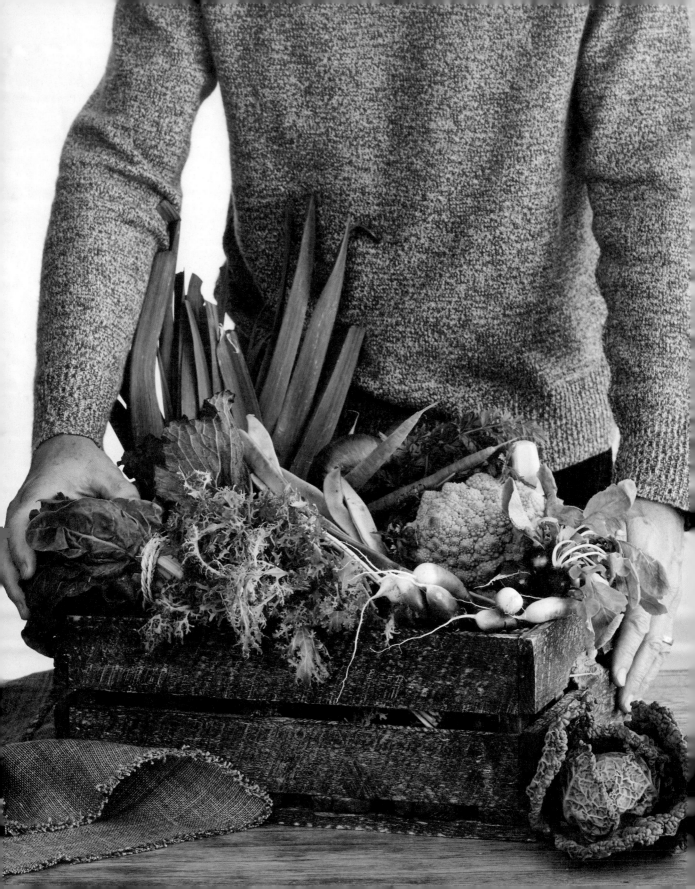

INTRODUCTION

I learned to love cooking in the 1970s, when many people thought Betty Crocker was a real woman. She was actually invented by the food industry to get mothers to incorporate processed food into home-cooked meals—remember "Just add one can of Campbell's Condensed Cream of Mushroom Soup to your casserole"? It was the era of Tang (the drink of the astronauts in the Apollo space missions), Fleischmann's margarine, and bright orange Kraft Macaroni and Cheese. And who could forget the TV dinners? My favorite thing to do after school was to heat up the meat-like substance, grainy mashed potatoes, and overcooked peas and carrots of a Swanson Salisbury Steak dinner, set up my TV dinner tray (yes, it was a thing), and watch Superman and Batman.

We weren't perfect, but despite the Western world slowly opting for convenience, in my house we were committed, for the most part, to eating fresh, real whole food. My mother made home-cooked meals with fresh ingredients from our suburban garden (a true anomaly at that time). She was taught by my deaf grandmother, Mary, to "buy fresh, eat fresh."

My mother, Ruth, who grew up in New York in the 1930s in a Jewish family, told us stories of our great-grandmother Fanny, who would buy a live carp every Passover and keep it in the bathtub until it was time to make fresh gefilte fish. My mother and father lived in Europe for eleven years just after

World War II. I was born in Barcelona and lived there until I was four years old, and I remember the smells and sounds of the food markets. Every day my mother would go to the local markets and buy *real food*—nothing processed, packaged, or wrapped in cellophane. There were no grocery stores, just little stands—a "farmers' market" before there was a name for such a thing. She brought that sensibility to the suburbs of Toronto, where I mostly grew up. Our backyard was a mini-farm with plum, apple, and pear trees and a beautiful vegetable garden. I loved that I could just walk outside for a snack. I absorbed cooking skills from my mother and ate whole foods before they were referred to as such. There was no soda, candy, or junk, except of course for Oreo and Chips Ahoy cookies—and my afterschool TV dinners!

For me, cooking has always been synonymous with community and connection. My earliest food-related memories are of learning how to make chicken soup on Friday nights and latkes (potato pancakes) for Hanukkah. My mother taught me the basic building blocks of cooking: how to crush garlic and peel onions, when to cook what so that everything would come out perfect at the same time. It is what humans have done for millennia—transmitting the skills of gathering, preparing, and making food in community from generation to generation.

When I went to college, I moved into a group house with seven other health-minded people (okay, we called them hippies in those days). We each had to make dinner for eight people one night a week. We ripped up our lawn and turned our whole backyard into a big garden where we composted our scraps. We won our school's composting and recycling of the year award (in 1979, before it was cool) and our prize was a three-gallon tub of Cornell ice cream! This was where I developed my culinary chops and honed the art of cooking: chopping, seasoning, sautéing, baking, roasting, designing menus, and creating plant-rich dishes that not only tasted good but were good for us. We made our own bread, yogurt (yes, we were hardcore), and even maple syrup from the old maple trees in front of our house. Every night we ate together, shared stories, and talked about what we were learning, breaking bread and building friendships that have lasted a lifetime. Food is medicine, but community is medicine too.

Most importantly, I learned how to eat well and eat real food without a lot of resources. In college and medical school, I had $300 a month to pay for rent, food, and entertainment. We went to farmers' markets, shopped in bulk, and made amazing meals from simple fresh ingredients. In my medical residency, I lived on $27,000 a year while supporting a wife and two children. Even thirty years ago, that wasn't much for a family of four. Still, we made home-cooked meals most days of the week and delighted in our time spent together making food and connecting over dinner. Family dinners were a priority, a time to stop, cook together, eat, talk, and connect.

My love affair with cooking grew out of my mother's commitment to buying, making, and eating real food; she found joy in making food for others, in seeing happiness on their faces as they ate yummy food in celebration of life, family, and community. Unfortunately, this is not the case for most people.

Today, the food industry has hijacked our kitchens, not by accident, but by design. It has rebranded cooking as a chore, a burden, drudgery. "You deserve a break today." Nonsense. It's a con job to get us to buy prepared, processed foods. Many of my patients report feeling too stressed and too tired to cook, and on the rare occasions when they have the energy to cook, more often than not they are confused about *what* to cook. They are victims of the food industry initiative to subvert the American kitchen (and increasingly, the global kitchen), and they are not alone. We now have two generations of Americans who do not know how to cook, who have swallowed Big Food's propaganda that cooking is a difficult, time-consuming, expensive, onerous chore from which only they can save us. It's a lie. Don't buy it. Cooking and eating food are essential acts that make us human and connect us to what is real and important: the earth, nature, family, and community. Preparing and cooking food, for me, has always been a source of joy, nourishment, connection, and exploration. And with a little practice and guidance, it can be for you as well.

Cooking simple, whole foods isn't actually all that time-consuming—it can take less than an hour a day. And it's not that expensive, either. Studies show that it costs about a dollar more per day to eat real, whole foods. And when you count the price society pays for processed food—the harm it brings to our health, economy, climate, and environment—it is clear that real, whole foods are the far less expensive choice, both for our wallets and our bodies.

Our world has evolved into a place where processed junk foods are ubiquitous and cheap, and real, whole foods have somehow become luxury items. With easily available cheap foods and so much confusion around food in general, it's no wonder people reach for what's easy. The system we have was not created by accident. It is the result of massive efforts by the food industry to confuse the public. The industry subverts legitimate science by funding biased studies and deploying them to adversely influence food policies set forth by our government; it funds public health institutions that were originally designed to protect us, making them ineffective and even dangerous; and it drives behavior and attitudes about food with tens of billions in food marketing. Our confusion about food is manufactured, and the system is rigged.

This is why I wrote my last book, *Food: What the Heck Should I Eat?* Way too many people are confused about what constitutes proper nutrition, and way too many people have been sold the idea that cheap, fast food benefits them by eliminating the question of what to eat—meanwhile it has been destroying public health. We're also up against huge disparities in food accessibility within our country: Many people lack the resources to buy the right foods—6,000 communities lack the ability to buy fresh foods and 20 million children start their morning without breakfast. Populations like these are really struggling.

On the other hand, 40 percent of Americans are obese and 70 percent are overweight. This inequality is only more frustrating when you consider that 40 percent of our food supply (about $480 million worth) is wasted and thrown into landfills, contributing to climate change. It's clear there is work to be done to level the playing field when it comes to providing healthy food and nutritional resources for people everywhere.

And then there are the never-ending diet trends, the black and white guidelines full of unsustainable rules for finding your ideal weight and getting that beach body you've always dreamed of. It's no wonder people become confused about what eating well really means. The research is so heavily influenced by industry (just $1.5 billion goes to independently funded studies, versus over $12 billion to industry-funded studies every year) that even I was confused. Until, that is, I dug into the studies: who funded them, how they were designed, what conclusions could accurately be drawn from them, and how they fit into the overall body of research.

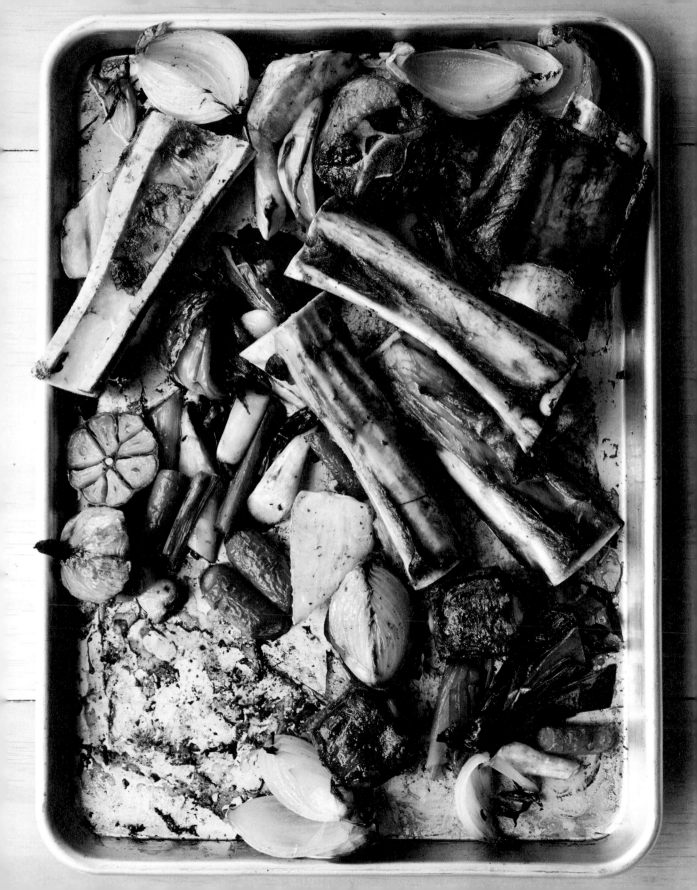

I've spent much of my career researching nutrition and experimenting with my own dietary framework. I wanted to fully understand the impacts of nutrition on a deeply personal level. Through decades of working with patients of all ages and in many states of health, I've seen the unique needs of the human body as well as its amazing ability to heal and regenerate when given the right food. It's astounding that the most important thing we need for a healthy, vibrant, successful life—how to care for and feed our bodies—is never taught in school. We're never taught to put the right kind of gas in our own tanks, but when we do it is powerful medicine that can keep us running at an incredible level.

The diet wars also drive confusion by framing concepts of Paleo, vegan, low-fat, low-carb, raw, keto, and more in opposition to each other. That's why I came up with the Pegan Diet—a mashup of Paleo and vegan—as a spoof on the extremism. While sitting on a panel at a medical conference, discussing the importance and discrepancies of modern nutrition, I found myself between one doctor who was a strict vegan and another who was passionately Paleo. Each had different views on why their diet was the one and only way to optimal health. When it was my turn to talk, I joked that the best description of my dietary beliefs must be "Pegan"—and the Pegan Diet was born.

I examined the concept and it actually made sense: a plant-rich diet of whole foods that are low-glycemic, rich in phytonutrients, good fats, fiber, and more. It is an inclusive, nutrient-dense, sustainable way of eating for life; it's fun and irresistible deliciousness.

Increasingly, consumers want transparency and authenticity. They want to eat food that helps them thrive and that is light on the planet by promoting sustainability and even helping reverse climate change. This consumer-driven food movement is growing and working to change food production, processing, and consumption patterns. Even Big Food companies are shifting their products, removing bad ingredients and trying to adapt (which can be hard for many).

It's not perfect but it's a step in the right direction, driven by consumers who are voting with their dollars and purchases. The choices we make at the market have a far bigger impact than you might imagine. For example, many large corporations listened to consumer pleas for genetically modified organisms (GMOs) to be labeled, and thus removed themselves from the association working to block that process. Our choices not only drive positive shifts in Big Food, they support local economies and help communities thrive while we reap the benefits in our own health. With a little bit of planning and some helpful hacks, you can make simple, nutritious Pegan meals at home that are delicious *and* affordable. This book will show you how. Eating real food may not always be as convenient as other, less healthy options, but how convenient is illness and the cost of drugs, medical care, and disability? Hospital and medical bills are the number one cause of bankruptcy and many crowdfunding platforms are used to help struggling people pay their medical bills.

Most of the diseases that land people in the hospital or cause suffering and disability are lifestyle diseases. But lifestyle can also prevent and treat chronic disease. Food is more powerful than any drug when it comes to reversing disease (in fact, most drugs don't prevent disease, they merely manage it). Most diseases associated with aging are driven by food (bad food), but good food can often cure them.

One sixty-five-year-old woman in one of our Functioning for Life groups (at the Center for Functional Medicine) had type 2 diabetes and had been on insulin for ten years, plus she had heart failure, early kidney and liver failure, high blood pressure, and was morbidly obese. After three days of eating real food, she was off her insulin. After three months, she'd lost 43 pounds, reversed her heart failure, improved her kidney and liver function, and gotten off all her medications. After six months, she'd lost 63 pounds and counting. Good nutrition is not only about avoiding disease later, but about thriving now. Most of us don't know how bad we feel until we start to take care of ourselves and feed our bodies nourishing whole foods. The truth is that the key to a vibrant, thriving, happy, successful life, the foundation that will help us have energy, focus, and the ability to be present in our lives, starts at the end of our fork and in our kitchens.

If I had one "medicine" to take with me anywhere in the world to heal people it would be food. My patients are often shocked and surprised when their "incurable illnesses" are healed by a change in diet. It seems almost magical. But real food contains thousands of molecules, each designed to regulate and optimize the functions of your body—your gene expression, hormones, brain chemistry, immune system, gut microbiome, and more.

Let that sink in.

But food matters in ways that go far beyond personal health. Promoting the consumption of real whole foods can help us reverse America's epidemic of chronic disease and end the burden it puts on our economy and government (imagine if we had $3.4 billion more every year for programs that uplift communities and society). Eating the right foods can also address social justice issues, poverty, violence, educational gaps in learning, and even national security (70 percent of our military recruits are not fit to fight because of poor fitness). And eating food grown in ways that restores soil and sequesters carbon can help us contribute to the fight against climate change. We can change the world we live in by eating "food," not food-like substances, and we can improve the health of future generations and our planet in the process.

Last but not least, food brings us together. The simple acts of shopping, chopping, cooking, and eating have for centuries been at the center of human communities, whether it was the family, tribe, village, or neighborhood. I've had patients come in who are doing everything right—eating well, exercising, managing stress—but they are socially isolated and alone. As humans we crave connection, understanding, and the feeling of belonging. I believe food is a vital piece in helping us all achieve a sense of community in our own lives, and I hope you'll use this book to cultivate that through joyful and delicious gatherings. Create dinners for friends at home, have them help cook or bring their own homemade dishes for a potluck. Maybe create theme-based supper clubs for deep conversations about things that matter.

We have been brainwashed to think cooking is difficult, time consuming, and expensive. That's a lie propagated by the food industry. And now with wholesale stores and discounted retail whole foods companies like Thrive Market, cooking real food is affordable—all you need is a little practice. Cooking skills are an essential but a lost art. If you're rusty, or just learning how to cook, using recipes like those in this book can help you learn the basics: how ingredients work together, how to add them in the right order and get the timing just right. Knife skills, sautéing, baking, and roasting can be learned very quickly. If you have a body, cooking is as important for your health as brushing your teeth or cutting your fingernails. Take the time to cultivate culinary skills, be creative, have fun, put on happy music, and invite your friends, family, and kids to participate. The average person spends eight hours a day staring at screens. Cooking is a real activity, so get your hands messy, touch it, feel it, understand it, experiment, and try new things.

Let this book be your go-to guide for making food that looks good, tastes good, smells good, and is good for you. Let it help you bring people you love, or people you'd like to get to know better, together over tasty meals and inspiring conversation. Cooking is a revolutionary act, one that can heal you, your community, and even the planet. We have the power to change our world one bite at a time.

Wishing you health and happiness,
Mark Hyman, MD

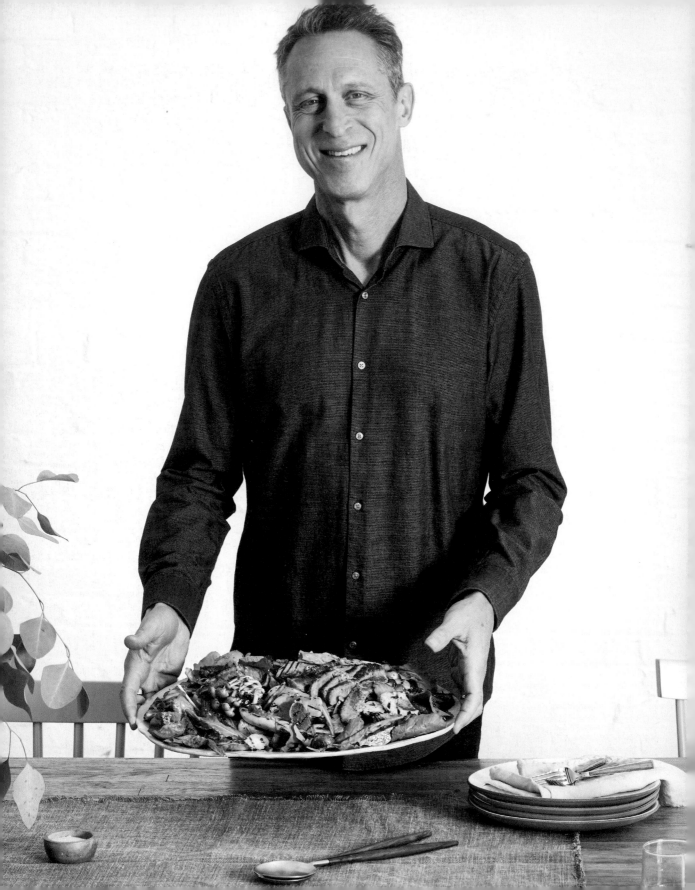

Part I

Learning
How to Eat

MY FOOD PHILOSOPHY

Food is a fundamental part of life, a need every human has in common with every other human. It's our fuel, yes, but it is so much more. It is information that transforms our biology with every bite, activating our potential for healing or creating imbalance that causes disease. Real, whole food contains biological instructions that promote health. It can optimize your gene expression, balance hormones, reduce inflammation, enhance brain function, and even improve the microbiome—the critically important ecosystem of bacteria in our gut. Our bodies perform all of these amazing functions with little to no conscious thought on our part. Food is the most powerful tool we have to take control of our health. Choosing the wrong foods leads us down a road of chronic disease, while choosing the right ones prevents illness and can even cure it.

Food is also very personal, and it means different things to each of us. We each have our very own food philosophy, a set of dietary principles that, consciously or not, dictate our daily choices. The way we choose to eat not only reflects the level of care we have for our health, it reflects the level of care we have for other humans, animals, and the environment. Every bite of food is a vote. We vote for our health, our communities, our farmers, our environment, our climate, and even the health of our economy. Food is connected to almost everything that matters to us.

Still, many of us are confused about what to eat. The science seems to be all over the place. Vegan, Paleo, keto, high-carb, low-carb, low-fat, high-fat, lectin-free, flexitarian, raw foods, and on and on. What's an eater to do? The good news is there are some commonsense nutritional principles, backed by good science, on which most experts agree (believe it or not).

The truth is, there is more agreement than disagreement about the healthiest way to eat. This cookbook is your road map to ending nutritional whiplash. It is full of practical guidance on what and how to eat based on scientific data infused with common sense. The recipes are yummy, nourishing, and easy to prepare, and they will help you and your family thrive.

The Social Implications of Food

Food is not just a tasty morsel at the end of your fork. It connects you to almost everything that matters: the soil in which it was grown or raised, the health of our climate and environment, the humans who helped grow it, the humans along the supply chain from field to fork, and our nation's public health status and economy. It even relates to our children's ability to focus and learn at school.

Food is a deeply personal choice, but it is also profoundly political. Our food purchases matter. Imagine if for one day the whole world ate nothing processed—no fast food, only organic or regenerative whole foods cooked at home with love and community. Big Food and policy makers would take notice. The collective food movement has already affected big companies. For example, the public outcry over GMO labeling and Big Food lobbyists influenced some of the biggest food companies (Nestlé, Unilever, Danone, Mars) to quit the Grocery Manufacturers of America because they were obstructing GMO labeling efforts and other important policies to improve the food system.

Our current federal food policies encourage Big Food to put private profit over public health. Despite the food system being the biggest national and global industry (over $1 trillion in the US and $18 trillion a year globally), we have no integrated, coordinated set of food policies. In fact, we have many agencies governing our food system, and their goals are often at odds with each other.

For example, the government tells us to eat five to nine servings of fruits and veggies a day. Fruits and vegetables are known as "specialty crops," and they receive just 1 percent of the more than $25 billion the United States Department of Agriculture (USDA) spends to support agriculture. The other 99 percent of the USDA's current funding goes to support commodities (corn, wheat, soy, etc.); those government subsidy–supported crops are turned into processed, high-sugar, high-glycemic, toxic, industrial foods that have been proven to increase chronic disease and death and which our dietary guidelines tell us to avoid. If we all followed our government's advice to eat five to nine servings of fruits and vegetables each day, 50 percent of our diet should be fruits and vegetables and plant foods. Yet only 2 percent of our agricultural land is used for these crops, while 59 percent is used to grow commodity crops, the raw materials for processed food. And if USDA subsidies were designed with the government's dietary recommendations in mind, a much larger percentage of the funding would support the production of healthy fruits and veggies instead of commodities destined to become junk food. Plus, we spend about $85 billion through our food stamp program (SNAP), most of which goes to pay for processed food, including over 30 billion servings of soda for the poor every year.

Then Medicaid and Medicare pick up the tab for chronic diseases that our misaligned government policies create. This sounds crazy, but it's true—and it's only one example. Instead of throwing up our hands, my colleague Dariush Mozaffarian, the dean of the Friedman School of Nutrition Science and Policy at Tufts University, and I took action to change this. We worked with an enlightened congressman, Tim Ryan of Ohio, who, along with one of his colleagues, requested that the Government Accountability Office, an independent arm of Congress that evaluates the effectiveness and economic impact of government policies, review all of America's food-related government policies and make recommendations for change. It won't solve everything, but it will make the problem clear.

Currently, obesity and type 2 diabetes account for $3.4 trillion a year in direct and indirect medical costs, or almost 20 percent of our entire economy. This epidemic of diabesity is blamed on individuals: It's a matter of personal responsibility, people say. Just eat less and exercise more. It's a lack of willpower, a personal failure. In the face of a toxic nutritional environment jam-packed with foods designed to be addictive, relying on willpower to stay healthy is like using a thimble to bail water out of a sinking ship. What we eat is a result of what is grown, made, advertised, and sold.

Let's take a deeper look at the implications of our current food policies. Unregulated food marketing targets children and minorities. The result? Escalating childhood obesity, chronic disease, and dramatic racial disparities when it comes to health, predominantly in the African American and Latino communities.[1] This has created an achievement gap wherein obese children perform more poorly in school than their healthier classmates. The processed, industrial diet has been shown to perpetuate poverty and chronic disease, impair brain function, and even drive violence and crime.[2]

But what about the US Dietary Guidelines? Shouldn't they be guiding our health in the right direction? Yes, they should, but they're not. Rather than reflecting science, they are heavily influenced by the Big Food lobby. For example, there is no scientific data to support the recommendations that adults drink three glasses of milk a day and that kids drink two, yet our guidelines demand that school lunches include milk. And to make matters worse, they don't even recommend whole milk; they encourage children to consume low-fat, flavored, sweetened milk that contains nearly as much sugar as a soda. But the jig may finally be up.

In 2017, as a result of the dogged persistence of Nina Teicholz, a one-woman lobbying force, Congress mandated that the National Academy of Sciences review the US Dietary Guidelines. They found that the Dietary Guidelines Advisory Committee had not only ignored significant scientific findings, it was also hobbled by significant conflicts of interest stemming from members' ties to the food industry. For example, important research showing that saturated fat is not connected to heart disease and that cereal grains can have harmful effects was never even reviewed.

We're not given a fair chance to make our own decisions around food. Our food labeling system is confusing, and while certain changes have been made, like the use of "Added Sugars" in nutrition information, nothing about this framework earnestly pushes consumers to buy real, nutrient-dense items like fruits and vegetables. Instead, it has them focus on single nutrients such as saturated fat or sugar and gives the food industry the ability to dial up or down ingredients rather than sell us whole, real food.[3]

Industrial animal agriculture, also known as concentrated animal feeding operations (CAFOs), creates multiple layers of destruction: It's inhumane for the animals; it destroys the environment through the use of petroleum-based fertilizers, pesticides, and herbicides; it is a major contributor to climate change from soil destruction and methane production;[4] and it creates antibiotic-resistant superbugs from the overuse of antibiotics in animal feed used to promote growth and reduce infection from overcrowding.

All of this keeps us sick and fat and weighs heavily on the economy. We have an escalating federal debt due in large part to the fiscal burden of chronic disease on Medicare and Medicaid, much of which could be prevented with proper nutrition and lifestyle choices. Science confirms that poor diet can create poverty, violence, and social injustice due to its effects on behavior. I once had a prison inmate write to me, telling me how his whole world changed when he changed his diet. He no longer had the angry, violent outbursts that had led to his crime, and science supports his story—studies have shown feeding prisoners healthy diets can reduce crime among inmates by 56 percent.[5] This represents yet another way our economic burden could be lessened by the power of real, nutritious foods.

There is so much more hiding in our food than we're led to believe—and I'm not just talking about ingredients. The social implications of what we eat run wide and deep. Our food policies do not support public health. They create a wellness deficit early in life for our most fragile humans, take advantage of low-income families, and perpetuate a "sick care"—rather than a health care—system. What we put on our fork at every meal has the power to transform our health and the economy, reverse climate change and environmental damage, and help reduce poverty, violence, social injustice, and more.

These principles form the pillars of a Pegan Diet and are a guide (not a rigid prescription) to a way of eating that supports you and the world around you.

What It Means to Go Pegan

My own journey sifting through nutritional literature and getting caught in the middle of the nutrition wars led me to create the Pegan Diet. It represents a middle ground based on science and is infused with common sense that accommodates a wide variety of eating styles and preferences while doing good for your taste buds, your body, the earth, and our society.

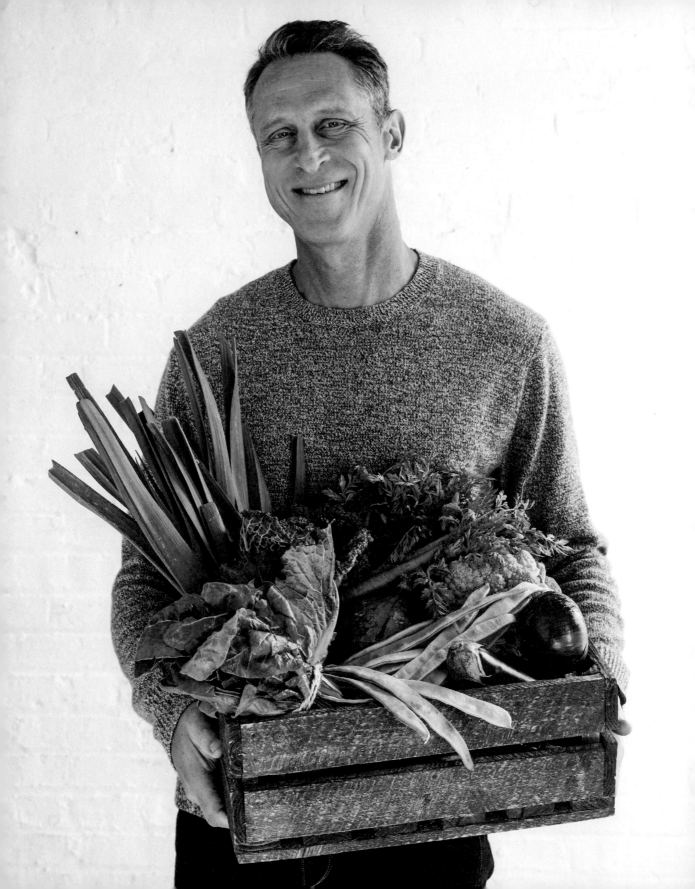

My food philosophy, based on nutritional research, recognizes the beneficial aspects of vegan and Paleo diets, and many other types of diets, too. In fact, there are beneficial commonalities between these seemingly polarized diets; there are also aspects that make neither of them completely optimal on their own. That's why I used the most well-researched and supported nutritional principles to create my Pegan approach, and I have seen its amazing impacts firsthand. Best of all, there is room for personalization within it.

To understand the benefits of the Pegan Diet, let's start by looking at the basic principles and similarities of the vegan and Paleo diets.

The Vegan Diet: All Plants, All the Time

The vegan diet revolves around avoiding any animal products whatsoever—meat, dairy, eggs, and other animal by-products like honey, though not all vegans are so strict they avoid the latter. Some people practice veganism for moral reasons while others believe it is best for their health. The ideal form of this diet would involve plenty of whole, plant-based foods. Unfortunately, it's possible to be vegan and eat a diet filled solely with highly refined grains and sugars, genetically modified soy, and other processed foods with artificial ingredients and additives. With the villainization of meat, most people eating this way thought they were making healthy choices based on what their diet didn't contain, instead of thinking about the ingredients that it did.

Another concern with the vegan diet is that it doesn't provide enough of the essential omega-3 fatty acids DHA and EPA, both of which are necessary for optimal health due to their role in balancing inflammation, the root of all chronic disease. They are also vital for good brain function and play a host of other supportive roles in the body. Additionally, vegans are at a greater risk for deficiencies in vitamin B_{12}, iron, zinc, and vitamin D, since they avoid the foods that naturally contain these nutrients, so supplementation is necessary.[6]

And then there is the great protein debate. Yes, vegans can get complete proteins by combining plant-based sources like beans, grains, nuts, and legumes; however, this is hard to do and often still leaves them short on essential amino acids. Getting enough protein from these sources also comes with a shocking amount of carbohydrates. It takes 3 cups of beans to get the amount of protein from a 6-ounce piece of chicken. And those 3 cups of beans contain a whopping 348 grams of carbs (although a good portion come from fiber), compared to 0 grams carbs in the chicken. Considering that 70 percent of Americans are overweight and 50 percent have pre-diabetes or type 2 diabetes, high-carbohydrate diets are a big problem.

The upside of veganism, when practiced correctly, is that eating wholesome plant-based foods provides many other vitamins, minerals, phytonutrients, antioxidants, fiber, and healthy fats while avoiding the toxicity of feedlot meat and dairy products, as well as the inhumane treatment of animals. The hormones, antibiotics, poor living conditions, and unnatural diets of conventionally raised animals greatly and negatively affect the quality of their meat, eggs, and milk—passing problems on to those who eat them.

Vegans avoid this issue altogether. However, the moral, ethical, and environmental issues related to eating animal products are very different than the health issues. They often get conflated and mixed up. On the health side, there are concerns about veganism because the notion that it is the best diet for humans is only supported by data that is inconclusive at best. It is certainly better than a processed, industrial diet, vegan or otherwise, but it may not be the best long-term diet for humans. To dig deeper into the science around these questions, I encourage you to read my last book, *Food: What the Heck Should I Eat?*

The Paleo Diet: Eating Like Our Ancestors

Now, let's turn the tables and look at what it means to eat Paleo. This diet is based on the idea that our bodies are best acclimated to the foods that existed in the Paleolithic era, before the birth of agriculture. The foods that were most commonly available to our ancestors at the time were wild meats and fish; whole, nonstarchy vegetables; certain starchy high-fiber root vegetables and wild winter squashes; and small amounts of seasonal fruit as well as nuts and seeds. Sugar intake was extremely low, except for the sugar naturally occurring in fruit and possibly small amounts of honey. This diet excludes grains, dairy, legumes and beans, and other types of sugar because humans in the Paleo era hadn't yet figured out how to cultivate these crops. We relied on foraging as a means for survival. Because of this, we only ate meat and fish when we were able to catch it; meaning we ate animal products in their cleanest and wildest forms and in much smaller amounts than we do now.

The Paleo diet is generally low-glycemic and helpful for blood sugar regulation.[7] It also puts a heavy emphasis on quality—meaning organic and seasonal vegetables, grass-fed and pasture-raised animal products, and wild-caught fish. A downfall of the modern Paleo approach, though, is that meat has become the cornerstone of the diet for many, despite the fact that it wasn't even close to as widely available to humans in the Paleolithic era as it is now. There was actually a huge amount of fibrous plant foods in our ancestors' diet, providing between 100 to 150 grams of fiber per day, compared to the current daily average of 8 to 15 grams. And packaged "Paleo friendly" foods are popping up everywhere—turning the entire concept of eating closest to the earth on its head.

The ideal version of the modern Paleo diet would look something like this: lots of nonstarchy vegetables; small amounts of low-glycemic fruits; grass-fed meat or pasture-raised poultry as a complementary part of the meal (not the star); some fatty, wild-caught, low-mercury fish and pastured eggs; a decent amount of healthy fats like olives, olive oil, avocado, coconut oil, nuts, and seeds; and the occasional use of honey and other minimally processed sweeteners like maple syrup in small amounts.

The Pegan Diet: A Synthesis of Science and Common Sense

The only real difference between vegan and Paleo is whether you eat animal products versus beans and grains as the source of your protein. Otherwise they are nearly identical. The most ideal version of each involves lots of wholesome, unprocessed plant foods. Paleo is generally higher in protein, vitamin B12, and other micronutrients than the vegan diet, but the vegan diet may be richer in fiber and antioxidants compared to the meat-heavy approach that some advocates of Paleo take today. After trying each of these diets myself, I've settled on a happy medium, combining the best parts of each with concepts from other diets and the anti-inflammatory and detoxification principles of functional medicine to create the balanced, inclusive Pegan Diet. This diet has not only drastically changed many of my patients' lives by leading them to vibrant health, but it's done the same for my own as well. For some patients I will make modifications based on metabolism, gut health, autoimmune disease, and more, but always using food as medicine.

I've organized the Pegan Diet into ten principles to provide a big picture of the steps you can take to change your diet right away. This way of eating is not meant to be a quick fix or crash diet—those words have no place in the vocabulary of someone pursuing long-term health. The Pegan Diet is a lifestyle; it's a food philosophy, not a diet. It provides guidelines that you can live by and thrive by. I recommend you eat this way every day to feel your best.

The Ten Principles of a Pegan Diet

1. Plants Should Be the Star of Your Diet

This is the simplest, most effective way to turn your health around. I call this a plant-rich diet rather than exclusively plant-based. More than half your plate, ideally 75 percent of it, should be filled with veggies *at every meal*. The deeper and more diverse the color the better. Eating a rainbow of colors every day is a surefire way to get an abundance of nutrients and beneficial phytochemicals through your diet. Stick with mostly nonstarchy varieties (for example leafy greens, cucumbers, celery, cauliflower, peppers, radishes, etc.) to support healthy blood sugar and insulin response. These foods are high in fiber, too, so they'll fill you up without filling you out. Limit starchier options, especially big starchy potatoes (the small fingerling or Peruvian heirloom potatoes are fine in moderation). Also enjoy but limit winter squash and sweet potatoes to no more than ½ cup per day. And don't forget—French fries and ketchup don't count as vegetables! This is a lie we've been told by the food industry (via our government policies)—don't be fooled. Always choose real vegetables in their most whole and natural form.

2. Quality Counts, in More Ways Than One

This means pesticides, antibiotics, hormones, GMOs, additives, preservatives, dyes, artificial sweeteners, and any other chemicals or fake food-like ingredients need to be avoided. In fact, many food additives that are banned in Europe are allowed in the US, including potassium bromate and azodicarbonamide (found in yoga mats and, at one point, Subway sandwiches). Other banned additives allowed in the US are BHA and BHT (why would anyone want to add something called butylated hydroxytoluene to their food?), brominated vegetable oil, Yellow Dyes (or should I say "dies") Nos. 5 and 6, Red Dye No. 40, and many farm animal drugs including bovine growth hormone (for dairy cows), and ractopamine (used for growth). Oh, and by

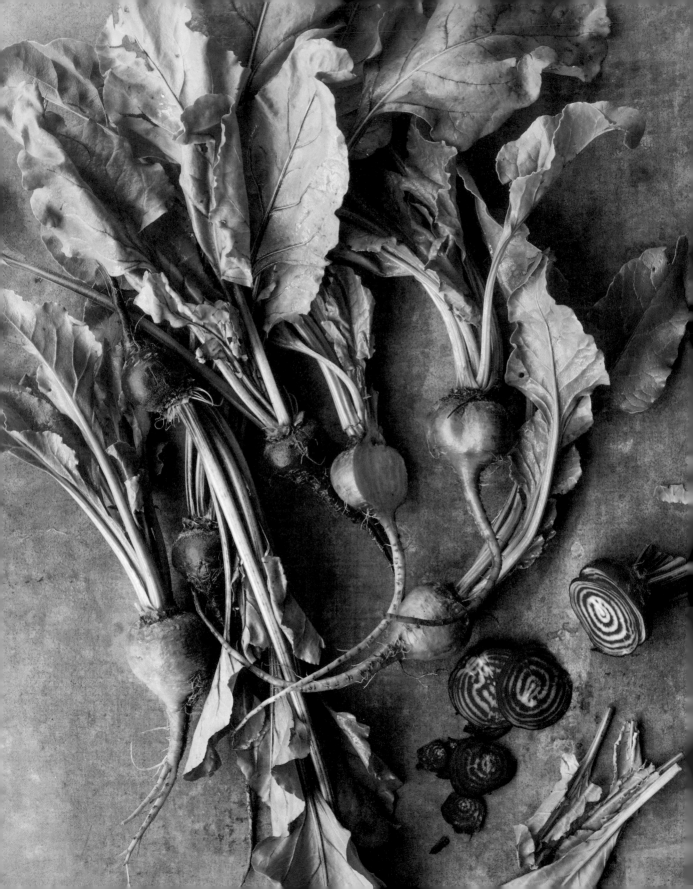

the way, Europe has pretty much banned most GMO foods.

These food-like substances may create problems in many ways—they may be carcinogenic, affect brain chemistry and behavior, cause weight gain, or create allergies, leaky gut, and more. It's best to limit all packaged goods as much as possible and instead choose natural foods that don't require a box or bag as often as you can. An avocado doesn't require a label—neither does a bunch of kale or a pint of fresh strawberries from the farmers' market.

In my opinion, we should avoid genetically modified food as much as possible. The jury is still out, but I prefer to practice the "precautionary principle," otherwise known as "better safe than sorry." This is a large uncontrolled experiment on the human population, just like the invention of Crisco and trans fats, which we used for a hundred years before it was "discovered" that they kill hundreds of thousands of people a year and were declared not safe to eat and banned as a food additive.

For the packaged items you do end up buying, be sure to read each and every label. Basically, if a product contains an ingredient that you don't have in your cupboard and wouldn't use in home cooking, then don't buy it. You might think, "Oh, it's just small amounts, it couldn't hurt." If only that were true. We consume an average of 3 to 5 pounds of a variety of 3,000 food additives every year! When considering purchasing packaged food, ask yourself: Are there fewer than five ingredients? If it's an animal product, was it raised or produced as close to its wild and natural state as possible? If you answer any of these questions with a "No," choose something else. The choice is always yours to make.

3. Go Gluten-Free or Gluten-Light, and Avoid or Limit Most Dairy

Going gluten-free is not just a fad, it's actually better for our health. In fact, gluten (the protein in wheat, rye, and barley) has been found to damage the lining of the gut, even in those who aren't considered sensitive to gluten and show zero symptoms of intolerance.[8] Our bodies just don't know what to do with it, so it can confuse the immune system and set off a cascade of health problems. Plus, most industrial wheat is sprayed with glyphosate (also known as Roundup) at harvest to exfoliate the plant, making the wheat easier to harvest—this is why breakfast cereals have high levels of glyphosate. A little Roundup with your Cheerios for breakfast?

The other reason to limit gluten is that almost no one eats wheat berries or true whole wheat. It is eaten as refined white flour. And don't think products advertised as whole wheat are any better. Unless your bread is made from unground wheat berries, it acts just like sugar in your body. Below the neck, your body can't tell if you just ate a bagel or a bowl of sugar. Eliminating gluten can have profound positive health impacts: reduced inflammation, weight loss, better gut health, and more. The only way to know for sure if gluten is affecting you is to stop eating it for a month and see how different you feel. That's better than any test or doctor or cookbook author telling you what's true!

Dairy is another food that just doesn't work for most people. It's nature's perfect food for a calf, not a human. Some 75 percent of the human population is lactose intolerant. Dairy has more than sixty naturally occurring hormones that can cause cancer and weight gain, and low-fat versions are even worse.[9] Limit dairy as much as possible, and if you're going to indulge, look for full-fat options from grass-fed cows. Sheep and goat dairy products may be better tolerated and less inflammatory than cow dairy because they contain A2 casein, not the gut disturbing, inflammatory A1 type found in conventional cow dairy. Ghee, however, which is clarified butter that has had the milk proteins removed, is often well tolerated and is a healthy, stable fat for cooking.

4. Limit Gluten-Free Grains, Too

Despite the fact that they're gluten-free, many grains still raise blood sugar. Stick with low-glycemic options, what I like to call "weird" grains or non-grain grains such as black rice, millet, quinoa, teff, buckwheat, and amaranth, and limit portions to no more than ½ cup per meal. White rice can actually be well-tolerated by some people when it's cooked and then chilled, which allows resistant starch to form. This starch is not absorbed and digested, so it doesn't cause a rise in blood sugar. It also has the added benefit of feeding good gut bacteria.

Oats are technically gluten-free, but they're commonly cross-contaminated with gluten and can also have a more severe impact on blood sugar and stress hormones than other grains. Plus, they have been found to make people hungrier,[10] so I suggest avoiding them. Some studies show that even gluten-free oats may contain gluten. Clinically speaking, my gluten sensitive patients don't get better until they get rid of oats, too.

And then there are the many gluten-free products on the market these days. A word to the wise—don't trust them just because they're labeled gluten-free. Oftentimes, they are loaded with more sugar and artificial ingredients than the processed food they're aiming to replace. Gluten-free cookies and cake are still cookies and cake, and they may be even worse in terms of sugar content and glycemic index.

Another issue with grains of all kinds is that they may exacerbate auto-immunity and digestive issues. Anyone struggling with these issues, as well as type 2 diabetics, may be able to more effectively treat and even reverse their diseases by eliminating grains from their diet.

5. Avoid Sugar and Eat Fruit in Moderation

Of all of the changes that my patients make, the one that makes the fastest and most significant impact on their health is limiting or removing refined sugars. You should eat a diet low in anything that might spike blood sugar and increase insulin production, as these processes are linked to inflammation, obesity, diabetes, Alzheimer's, cancer, heart disease, stroke, infertility, and more. The evidence shows us that sugar's effects on our neurochemical pathways create addictive behavior like cravings, bingeing, and even withdrawal, and it has been found to increase dopamine, which mimics the effects of opiates.[11] In fact, sugar lights up the addiction center in the brain in the same way as heroin or cocaine.

Sugar, flour, and any type of refined carbohydrates should only be eaten on rare occasions. If you must sweeten something, choose small amounts of natural sweeteners that at least have some antioxidants, vitamins, and minerals in them, like date sugar, molasses, maple syrup, and raw honey. Fruits can contribute to rises in blood sugar, so it's best to go easy on them. However, certain choices are better than others. Aim for most of your fruit intake to be from low-glycemic options like berries, kiwis, pears, and nectarines, and save others, like pineapple, mango, and grapes, as an occasional treat. Think of dried fruit as candy and keep it to a minimum.

6. Eat Clean Meat, Poultry, and Whole Eggs

I like to use the phrase "condi-meat" when it comes to consuming animal protein—a healthy addition when eaten in small quantities, but it doesn't need to be the main course. Vegetables should always be the star of your meals and animal products should be consumed in servings of 4 to 6 ounces (and not necessarily at every meal). And no, eating meat won't clog your arteries, cause cancer, lead to type 2 diabetes, and take years off your life[12]— science has debunked these myths, and we can now look at meat as the nutrient-dense food that it really is. There is one caveat though: quality. We are what our meat eats. Factory farmed animals are fattened up with hormones, antibiotics, candy (yep, it's true—Skittles if you really want to know!), and poor-quality GMO grains grown with pesticides and herbicides. Consuming the meat of these unhealthy animals is not going to do your health or the environment any favors.

Animals that are fed a wholesome diet of the types of food they evolved to eat (grass), and are allowed to move freely, produce significantly healthier meat with higher concentrations of nutrients than conventionally raised meat, without the toxicity. Some suggest that regenerative agriculture—range feeding that mimics traditional herds of animals—can also restore topsoil, sequester carbon, and hold huge amounts of water, which prevents floods and droughts. If you are interested in this topic, read *Kiss the Ground* by Josh Tickell, or watch the movie (kisstheground.com).

When grocery shopping, look for grass-fed meat and pasture-raised poultry. When eating eggs, eat the whole thing! No need to discard the yolk, which contains many nutrients and will not negatively impact your cholesterol or cause heart disease as previously preached. And that's not only my opinion, it's actually part of our 2015 US Dietary Guidelines.[13] Just look for eggs that come from pasture-raised hens, which are richer in nutrients, and be wary of eggs boasting labels like "cage-free" and "vegetarian-fed," which could still be from hens in poor, cramped living conditions without adequate access to the outdoors and a proper diet.

7. Choose Low-Mercury, Sustainably Harvested Fish

When eating fish, always be sure to choose low-mercury and low-toxin varieties. Enjoy wild-caught salmon, mackerel, anchovies, sardines, and

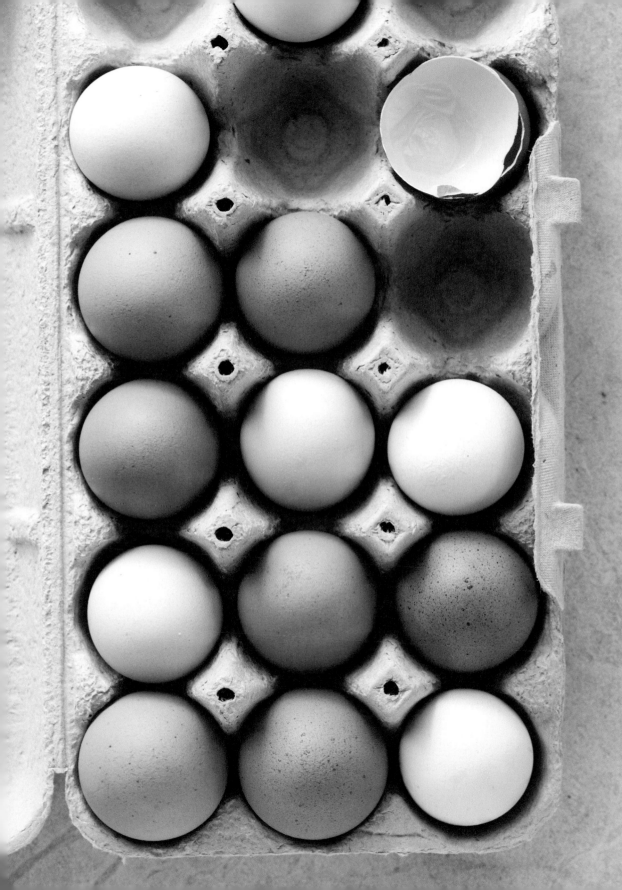

herring, or what I like to call SMASH fish. These species are high in omega-3s and lower in mercury than other options. Large fish are higher in the oceanic food chain, so they accumulate more mercury and toxins like PCBs. Clams, scallops, mussels, oysters, and Gulf shrimp are also healthy options to include in your Pegan Diet. Avoid swordfish, shark, marlin, grouper, king mackerel, Chilean sea bass, halibut, and tuna due to their higher levels of toxins. It's also important to go with seafood that has been sustainably harvested to avoid overfishing and bycatch.

8. Eat Lots of Healthy Fats

Yes, it's okay to eat fat! The catch is that you need to eat the right types. The low-fat diet craze made us sicker, fatter, and unhappier than ever before. It's no surprise, considering that fat is an essential macronutrient for our brains and bodies, providing structure, thermoregulation, hormone production, and so much more. We need to eat the right ones for optimal health—including saturated ones. Omega-3 fats from seafood, nuts, and seeds (not the fried, salted, or chocolate ones!), monounsaturated fats from olive oil and avocados, and saturated fats from coconut oil and coconut butter, whole eggs, sustainably raised or grass-fed meats, and even grass-fed butter or ghee—are all essential to a healthy and balanced diet.

9. Vegetable Oils Are Not a Health Food

Canola, sunflower, corn, grapeseed, safflower, peanut, sunflower, palm, soybean, and vegetable oils are inflammatory and abundant in fried and prepared foods. These are the fats you need to worry about, despite the fact that they were long promoted as health foods. And be sure to avoid anything that says "hydrogenated" or "partially hydrogenated," as those oils are made using a chemical process that converts vegetable oils like those listed above into solid fats (like margarine and vegetable shortening) for ease of use in packaged and prepared goods. This turns vegetable oils into trans fats, which are a health nightmare. The FDA declared them unsafe to eat and ordered food companies to remove them from processed food, but beware—they are still out there. These kinds of oils may negatively impact cholesterol, promote insulin resistance and inflammation, and increase the risk of cardiovascular disease. They are a highly refined "new to nature" food that have only been consumed for the last hundred years or so.

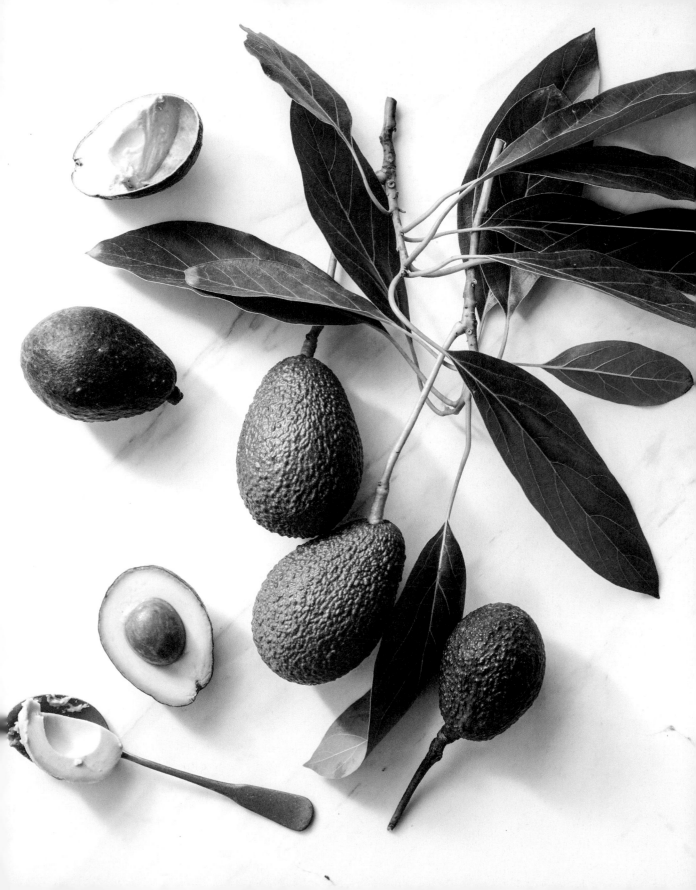

10. Enjoy Legumes Once in a While

The best legume options are lentils and peas, due to their lower starch content. And while beans can be a great source of fiber, protein, and minerals, they can also cause digestive upset. The lectins and phytates they contain may hinder mineral absorption, cause inflammation, and even exacerbate leaky gut and autoimmune disease.[14] However, there are ways to cook them to reduce these effects (soaking and pressure cooking). For these reasons, as well as their high-carbohydrate content, those with insulin resistance, type 2 diabetes, a sensitive gut, or autoimmune disease might do better avoiding legumes altogether. Everyone else may benefit from the vitamins, minerals, fiber, and resistant starch that can be found in legumes. Just limit servings to ½ cup once a day. Black beans, garbanzo beans, adzuki beans, and green beans are good options in addition to peas and lentils. And if you eat soy, always look for non-GMO, organic, fermented varieties.

The bottom line is this: I want you to eat real, whole foods. Sometimes that means following a recipe, and other times that means using what you have to make what you can. As you become more familiar with the Pegan Diet, shopping for the right foods and creating your own healthy meals will become second nature.

PEGAN FOOD PYRAMID

Recreational Treats
Sparingly

Gluten-Free Grains
Include ½ –1 cup of gluten-free whole grains per day

Fruits and Starchy Veggies
Focus on low-glycemic fruit, up to 1 cup per day, and up to ½ cup of starchy vegetables

Protein
Grass-fed meat, pasture-raised poultry and eggs, wild-caught low-mercury seafood, and beans, lentils, nuts, and seeds; 4 to 6 oz. of animal protein per day, up to 1 cup of legumes per day

Healthy Fats
3–5 servings per day, such as ½ an avocado or 1 tablespoon olive oil per serving

Non-Starchy Veggies, Herbs and Spices
Unlimited Amounts

RECIPE-FREE COOKING

I'm so excited to share all of the delicious recipes in this book with you, but I'm also excited to tell you more about my personal style of everyday cooking, one that becomes a natural skill once you get in the habit of preparing meals at home more often. I'm talking about recipe-free cooking.

Recipe-free cooking means you're able to look at what you have on hand and compose a snack or meal without having to plan ahead or even follow directions because you understand the way different flavors and textures work together. Throughout this book, I aim to help you get more familiar with the foods you should eat in abundance and those you should avoid. Recipes are a great way to build your kitchen confidence while getting to know these healthful foods, but before you know it, you'll be recipe-free cooking with ease.

My first rule of thumb for recipe-free cooking, and really any meal preparation for that matter, is that 75 percent of your plate by volume should be vegetables or plant foods, mostly nonstarchy ones. Think dark leafy greens, carrots, peppers, cauliflower, cucumbers, zucchini—there are so many options, you can make something new every night and never get bored. You just need a couple different kinds, hopefully with a range of colors, and you can plan the rest of your meal around them. Fresh herbs are another helpful component to create different flavor profiles in your meals.

Here are a few templates for my go-to meals that provide endless possibilities:

Berry Anything Smoothie

1 serving

Dairy-Free Milk: 8 ounces unsweetened dairy-free milk, such as coconut, almond, cashew, hemp, etc.

Frozen Berries: ½ cup blueberries, raspberries, strawberries, blackberries, or a combination

Greens: 1 large handful kale, spinach, or chard

Fat: 1 tablespoon nut or seed butter, such as almond, cashew, pecan, sunflower, or coconut

Optional add-ins: cacao powder, cacao nibs, cinnamon, pure vanilla extract, fresh ginger, fresh turmeric, unsweetened protein powder, MCT oil

Blend all ingredients until smooth and creamy.

Quick and Easy Super Salad

3 to 4 servings

Greens: 1 bunch kale or spinach, 1 head red leaf lettuce, or 1 bag arugula, rinsed and chopped

Veggies: As many nonstarchy ones as you'd like (peppers, radishes, cucumbers, onions, fennel, mushrooms, etc.), plus ½ to 1 cup of starchy varieties (like sweet potatoes or squash) if desired, chopped

Protein: 12 to 16 ounces of cooked wild-caught salmon or sardines; or cooked pasture-raised chicken, turkey, or grass-fed beef

Aromatics: 3 tablespoons chopped fresh parsley, cilantro, basil, oregano, mint, green onions, red onion, or shallots

Fat: 2 avocados plus 3 tablespoons of extra virgin olive oil

Acid: 3 to 4 tablespoons of fresh lemon or lime juice, red wine, balsamic, champagne, or apple cider vinegar

Toss all ingredients in a large bowl. Divide into three or four portions and serve.

Kitchen Sink Stir-Fry

4 servings

Fat: 2 tablespoons coconut or avocado oil

Aromatics: 1 yellow onion, 4 cloves garlic, and/or 1 tablespoon freshly grated ginger

Protein: 1 pound grass-fed ground beef, 1 pound pasture-raised chicken or turkey, or 8 ounces crumbled gluten-free tempeh

Veggies: 6 cups colorful mixed vegetables (think broccoli, peppers, mushrooms, carrots, cabbage, etc.)

Garnish: ¼ cup fresh lime juice or rice wine vinegar, 2 tablespoons coconut aminos or gluten-free tamari, ½ cup raw chopped cashews or almonds, fresh cilantro

Heat oil in a very large pan over medium heat. Add onions and sauté 2 to 3 minutes until onions are translucent, then add garlic and ginger and sauté another 2 minutes.

Turn heat to medium-high. Add protein and combine well with aromatics. Cook for 7 to 10 minutes until brown, breaking into pieces of the same size with a spatula while you cook.

Add vegetables and continue stirring and cooking for 5 minutes, until heated through but still crunchy.

Divide stir-fry between 4 bowls and top with desired garnishes.

Don't be afraid to get creative and try new things when you're cooking without recipes; that's often how some of the best meals come to be.

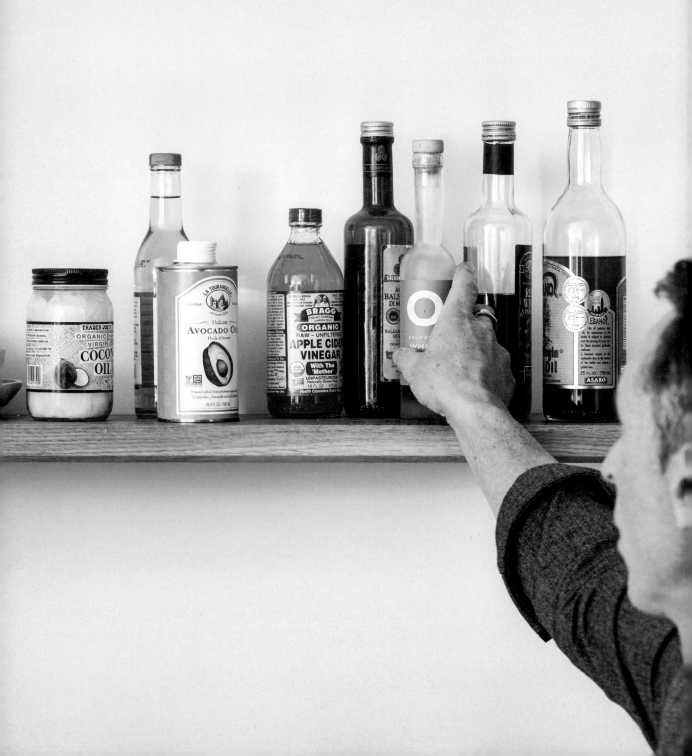

Part II

Creating a Conscious Kitchen

QUALITY OVER QUANTITY

Despite what many diets have preached over the past several decades, finding good health and a happy weight is not a matter of calories in and calories out.[1] If that were true, we'd all be at our ideal weight and obesity would be a thing of the past and not a growing epidemic. The number of calories you consume doesn't matter. What matters is how those calories affect your metabolism. The science shows that food is not just energy or calories, but information that regulates almost every function of the body. The "calories in, calories out" paradigm was developed by burning calories in a lab, which produces the same energetic results no matter the source. But this is not the case when you eat them. Why? Food contains much more than mere calories. It contains information that regulates hormones, genes, immune function, brain chemistry, the gut microbiome, and more. Your body is a complicated biochemical, hormonal soup controlled mostly by what you eat; the information in food can literally upgrade or downgrade your biological software with every bite.

Overcoming Calorie Counting

Do you think that 300 calories from an avocado have the same effect on your health as 300 calories from jelly beans? Of course not. There are different macronutrients (fat, protein, carbohydrates) and micronutrients (vitamins, minerals, antioxidants, phytochemicals) at play here. And the "information" in a Big Gulp or the equivalent amount of broccoli (both carbs) is profoundly different in quality and the impact on your health.

All calories are not created equal. That's why my approach to eating, the Pegan Diet, is all about focusing on quality and not quantity. When you eat whole, natural foods your body knows how to utilize their nutrients to keep you not just alive but thriving. It also means your body will naturally begin self-regulating the quantity of food you're consuming.

It's easy to overeat candy and junk food because those foods have been engineered by the food industry to keep you addicted; food scientists literally plot how to hijack your brain chemistry with the ingredients in their products by tapping into your "bliss point" and creating "heavy users." These are real terms food manufacturers use. On the other hand, your body knows when it's had enough real food because it can understand and properly metabolize the information it's been given. It feels physically full from fiber and nutrients. A simple principle is to ask yourself the question: Is this man-made or nature-made? It doesn't take a PhD in nutrition to figure that out and make a conscious choice about your next bite. Focus on real, whole food, on quality, and give up calorie counting. Your body will take care of the rest.

Choosing the Right Foods

While real, unprocessed, and minimally packaged foods are always my go-to, there are also many organic whole foods now available in packages, cans, and boxes, some of which can be helpful ingredients in healthy home cooking. If you truly want the Pegan Diet to bring your health to a new level, it's important to become a smart label reader.

When it comes to packaged foods, even those that you think are healthy, you need to read the full list of ingredients. Look for products with less than five ingredients, all of which you know and trust. Watch out for gluten's many aliases, such as wheat, barley, rye, spelt, bulgur, couscous, malt, and others. (See the Unsafe Gluten-Free Food List at celiac.com for a comprehensive list.) The same goes for sugar, which is also listed as corn syrup, cane juice, glucose, maltodextrin, fruit juice concentrate, and a variety of other names (more than sixty!). In general, anything ending in "-ose" is usually a sugar. There may be up to the equivalent of 33 teaspoons of sugar in the average bottle of ketchup, a great example of why reading labels is so essential to good health.

You also always want to look for preservatives, additives, artificial *and* natural flavors (neither are good), dyes, and flavor enhancers like monosodium glutamate (MSG), which also hides behind many names. Bottom line: Don't eat anything that contains ingredients you wouldn't have in your own pantry. And always beware of food marketing; it's designed to seduce you into an emotional purchase and may contain exaggerated claims. When in doubt, trust real foods that don't need a package or those with simple, identifiable ingredients.

Third-Party Labels and Certifications: Which Ones Really Matter?

Now that you better understand the benefits of a whole-foods diet, let's look at the many categories whole foods can fall into and which third-party labels you can trust.

ORGANIC

With the notable exception of seafood, the organic label can currently be applied to any type of food if it meets the designated criteria—although the USDA's National Organic Program (NOP) is currently in the process of developing organic practice standards for aquaculture.[2] Plants that are certified organic by a USDA-accredited agent are produced without genetic engineering, ionizing radiation, or sewage sludge, and are also free of many different types of chemical pesticides, herbicides, and synthetic fertilizers. Soil quality and certain physical, biological, and mechanical practices are also considered for organic certification. Produce can only be labeled organic if these many standards have been met and the land on which it was grown has been free from prohibited substances for three years before the time of harvest.

Many studies have linked organic vegetables to a decrease in negative effects from pesticides and have found that organic vegetables contain more nutrients and phytochemicals than conventional ones.[3] Studies in adults and children have linked pesticide exposure to cancer, as well as respiratory problems, depression, and even Parkinson's disease.[4] The Environmental Working Group has created two handy lists to help you prioritize which produce you should buy organic, if you have to choose. The Dirty Dozen tells you which foods are most highly contaminated with agricultural chemicals

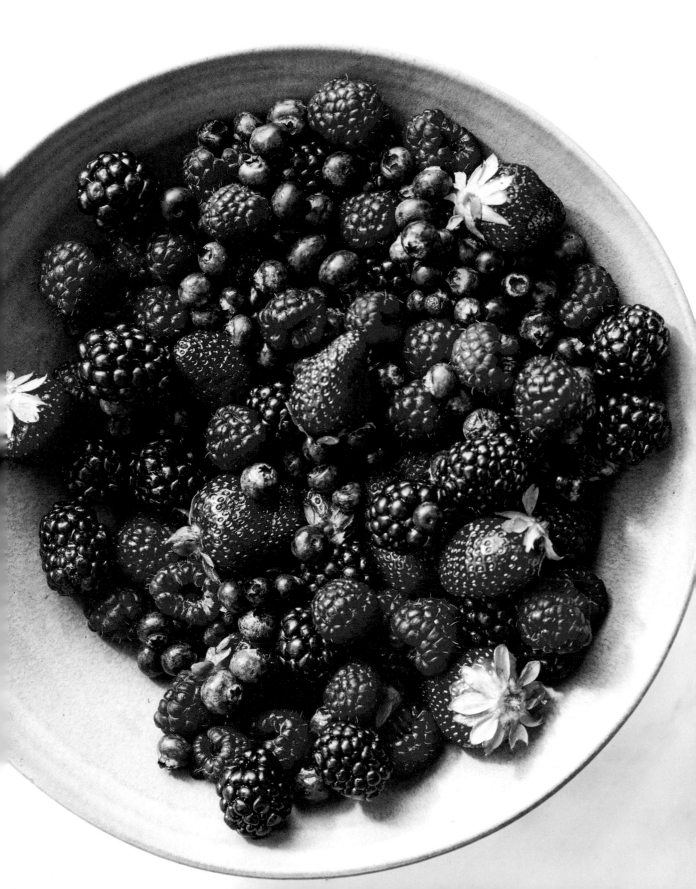

and the Clean Fifteen includes the foods with the least amount of contamination. (You can find the lists at ewg.org.)

NON-GMO

There's just not enough information out there about what GMOs (genetically modified organisms) are doing to our health. But the research and studies that are available do not make a positive case for these foods. Why take any chances with your health?

One way to avoid GMO foods is to buy organic. The only other way you can know for sure is to look for the Non-GMO Project Verified seal of approval. The Non-GMO Project is a nonprofit organization dedicated to educating consumers on alternatives to GMOs and advocating for the right to know what's in our food, down to the genetic level. When you see any product with the Non-GMO Project Verified seal, you can feel safe knowing you're avoiding genetically altered food, even if it's not organic. Many large companies use the Non-GMO Project as a certifying agency to label their products non-GMO, and, when you can't buy organic, this is the next best thing.

GRASS-FED OR PASTURE-RAISED

The label "grass-fed" is reserved for beef, bison, goat, lamb, sheep, and dairy products, while "pasture-raised" applies to pork, poultry, and eggs. These designations mean the product is from an animal that was raised eating its natural diet and foraging in the outdoors. This is the type of animal protein you want to consume. When a feedlot animal is eating candy (yep, this happens) or even when a cow exclusively eats corn (they're meant to eat grass), their bodies become inflamed, diseased, and overall unhappy. This is also why grass-fed and pasture-raised are a step above organic: A cow eating organic corn is still not eating its natural diet, though its meat is a much safer option than that of a cow pumped with antibiotics and fed GMO-corn.

WILD-CAUGHT AND SUSTAINABLY HARVESTED SEAFOOD

Wild-caught fish have greater nutritional value than farmed. Farmed fish have nearly undetectable amounts of beneficial omega-3 fatty acids, which are abundant in certain wild-caught fish like salmon and sardines. Many farmed fish are also fed corn and soy (very unnatural foods for a fish), creating higher levels of inflammatory omega-6 fatty acids that are passed on to you. Another downside to farmed fish is their higher levels of contaminants, like dioxins and polychlorinated biphenyls (PCBs). It's easy to see why wild-caught is better, but if farmed fish is your only option, look for those raised without antibiotics and hormones.

It's also important to source sustainably harvested seafood, which means methods were used to protect the ocean's natural supply and avoid harm to other sea life in the process. Natural Resources Defense Council, Clean Fish, Marine Stewardship Council, and the EWG are trustworthy resources for buying farmed and wild-caught seafood. And be sure to stick to the low-mercury varieties; in general, wild-caught salmon, mackerel, anchovies, sardines, and herring are your safest bets.

FAIR TRADE AND RAINFOREST ALLIANCE CERTIFIED

Food can have a cost much greater than its actual price. Some of the most common foods, like coffee, tea, sugar, and chocolate, are often produced by severely underpaid farmers and workers who are subjected to poor living conditions, little economic stability, and a lack of access to education within their communities. The Fair Trade Federation and World Fair Trade Organization are two groups with a deep commitment to supporting Fair Trade principles throughout the supply chain; you can find their logos on approved goods. And you can support sustainable farming practices by looking for the Rainforest Alliance seal when shopping; their logo means a product has been produced in a way that supports biodiversity conservation, effective planning and farm management systems, and sustainable and improved livelihoods for those involved in the growing and production processes.

Now you know how to make smarter decisions when it comes to reading labels. "Health washing," the practice of making a product seem healthy when it really is not, is alive and well in the world of food marketing. But the resources I've provided here will help you become a conscious consumer and see through the false claims of Big Food. Let's move on to more of the details involved in creating the right food environment for your home.

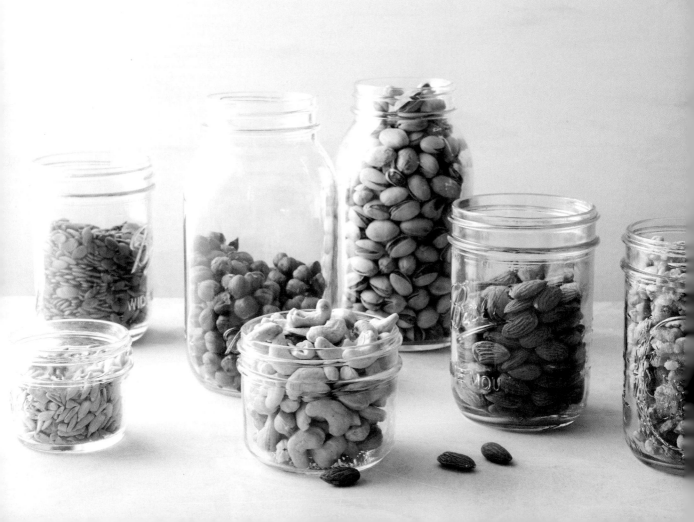

Stock Up

To make healthy eating a natural part of your lifestyle you need to set yourself up for success. Stock up on these wholesome ingredients so you can cook in confidence:

PANTRY STAPLES

- Seafood: canned wild-caught salmon, mackerel, sardines, anchovies
- Nuts: almonds, Brazil nuts, walnuts, pecans, macadamias, cashews, pine nuts, hazelnuts (all should be raw and unsalted)
- Seeds: pumpkin seeds, flaxseeds, hemp seeds, chia seeds
- Nut butters: almond, cashew, walnut, and pecan butter (without added oil, sugar, or salt)
- Oils: extra virgin olive oil, organic unrefined coconut oil (virgin or extra virgin), organic unrefined avocado oil (virgin or extra virgin)
- Vinegar: balsamic, apple cider, red or white wine, rice vinegar (but be sure to avoid added sugars)
- Sweeteners: unsulfured molasses, raw honey, maple syrup (use in small amounts)
- Whole grains: quinoa, millet, teff, amaranth, black rice, wild rice
- Legumes: smaller varieties like lentils, adzuki, navy beans
- Tea: Fair Trade organic green tea and hibiscus tea
- Chocolate: Fair Trade organic dark chocolate, at least 70 percent cacao (the higher cacao content and the less sugar, the better; eat only in moderation)
- Jerky made from grass-fed meat, pasture-raised poultry, or wild-caught fish (as long as there is no added sugar, preservatives, or other weird and unnecessary ingredients like gluten or MSG)

PERISHABLES

- Vegetables: organic, seasonal, nonstarchy vegetables; and organic, seasonal vegetables such as sweet potatoes and winter squash

- Fruit: organic, seasonal, low-glycemic fruit (especially berries, bonus points if they are wild, and frozen is okay!)
- Meat: grass-fed beef and lamb; pasture-raised pork and poultry
- Eggs: pasture-raised
- Seafood: wild-caught salmon and other SMASH fish (salmon, mackerel, anchovies, sardines, herring)
- Fats: grass-fed butter or ghee
- Tofu: organic and, if possible, sprouted
- Tempeh: organic, gluten-free
- Dairy: grass-fed yogurt or kefir from goat's or sheep's milk
- Hummus: organic (just be sure it's made with olive oil and without additives)
- Kimchi and sauerkraut: naturally fermented

CONDIMENTS
- Ketchup: organic and no sugar added
- Mustard: without added oils and additives
- Mayonnaise: made with avocado or olive oils
- Coconut aminos or gluten-free tamari: without sulfites, colorings, and sweeteners
- Chili sauce: avoid added chemicals and sulfites
- Miso: organic gluten-free
- Tahini: should only contain ground hulled sesame seeds

MEDICINAL SPICES AND HERBS
- Basil: good for the heart, antioxidant, antibacterial
- Black pepper: helps the absorption of nutrients
- Cayenne and all hot peppers: boost metabolism, increase circulation
- Cinnamon: improves circulation, antimicrobial

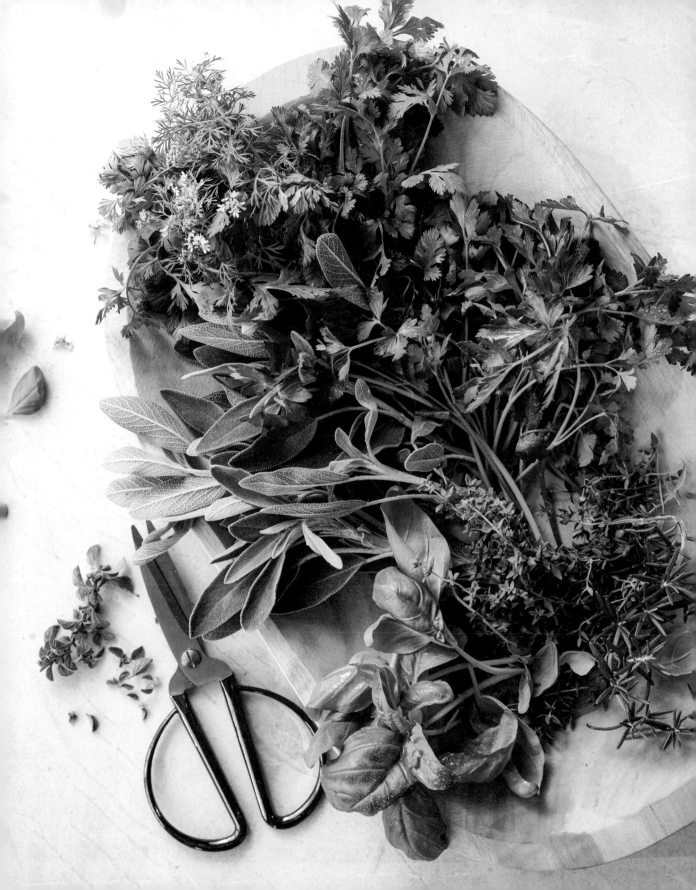

- Cloves: protect from environmental toxins, anticancer properties
- Coriander and cilantro: lower blood sugar, detoxifying
- Cumin: immune support, anticancer properties
- Ginger: helps digestion, anti-inflammatory
- Oregano: antimicrobial, antioxidant
- Parsley: promotes good breath, antioxidant, antitumor properties
- Rosemary: immune support, improves digestion
- Sage: brain support, anti-inflammatory, antioxidant
- Thyme: supports lung function, antioxidant, antibacterial
- Turmeric: benefits the heart, anti-inflammatory, anticancer properties

A NOTE ON SALT

While salt, or sodium more specifically, has been linked to hypertension, heart disease, and stroke, it's important to realize that this is only the case in a subset of people who are genetically salt-sensitive. Sodium is actually very important for our overall health, it just has to be in the right proportion to other minerals, particularly potassium. When the ratio of sodium to potassium gets out of balance, high blood pressure is the result. That's why we need to get the right amounts of each to stay healthy. Some of the best sources of potassium are cooked spinach, broccoli, squash, and avocados, while we can find naturally occurring sodium in meat, beets, carrots, celery, seaweed, and beans.

The table salt we've grown accustomed to in the US is highly refined; it's been stripped of any beneficial trace minerals and even has additives like anticaking agents and sugar. Instead, choose Himalayan pink salt, kosher salt, or sea salt. We can safely add these to our diet as long as we're also eating foods rich in potassium, though you still shouldn't overdo it. If you utilize the potent spices and herbs in the list above, you really won't need much salt to make your food taste good. Here's another tip: Add salt to your dishes after you're done cooking, you'll get more bang for your buck when it comes to flavor.

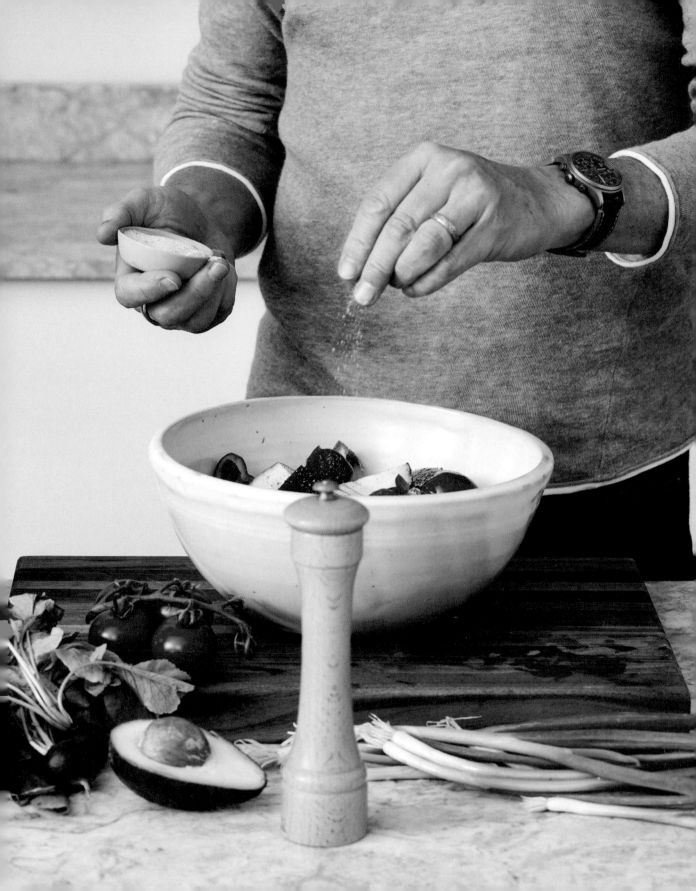

Eat the Rainbow

You'll hear me say this time and time again: Eat the rainbow. No, I don't mean sugary, artificially flavored, and colored candy. I'm talking about real, wholesome, brightly hued fruits and vegetables. If you want to use food as medicine, this is the simplest tip to follow. Our hunter-gatherer ancestors ate more than 800 varieties of plants, providing them with all of that fiber I mentioned earlier, along with an abundance of different nutrients. We should take a note from history and try to get as much diversity as we can in our diets, too.

Eat an assortment of colorful plant foods on a daily basis and you'll reap the benefits of numerous phytonutrients, vitamins, and minerals that support optimal health. The color of a plant signals different beneficial compounds within it, with each color group representing naturally protective and healing substances:

- *Blue-purple* signals the presence of anthocyanins in foods like eggplants, beets, blueberries, red cabbage, and purple potatoes. Anthocyanins have been found to prevent blood clots, delay cellular aging, and may even slow the onset of Alzheimer's.

- *Green* indicates the presence of phytochemicals like sulforaphane, isocyanates, and indoles, which are anticarcinogenic and detoxifying. Many green veggies are part of the *Brassica* family, which includes broccoli, Brussels sprouts, bok choy, arugula, kale, cauliflower, and more.

- *Orange* means the compounds alpha-carotene and beta-carotene are present and can be seen in foods like carrots, pumpkin, acorn squash, and sweet potatoes. Alpha-carotene protects against cancer and benefits skin and eye health; beta-carotene is a precursor to vitamin A and antioxidant within the body.

- *Pale green-white* is caused by compounds called allicins, which have powerful anticancer, antitumor, immune-boosting, and antimicrobial properties. These are present in garlic, onions, leeks, and others. Many of these same foods contain antioxidant flavonoids like quercetin and kaempferol.

- *Red* indicates a carotenoid called lycopene, found in tomatoes, bell peppers, and carrots. Asparagus also actually contains a good amount of lycopene—proof that you can't always judge a book by its cover. Lycopene is protective against heart disease and cancer due to its powerful antioxidant activity.

- *Yellow-green* means a food contains the carotenoids lutein and zeaxanthin, which are especially beneficial for the eyes and help protect the heart against atherosclerosis. Vegetables in this group may not always appear yellowish. In addition to yellow summer squash and orange bell peppers, spinach, collard greens, mustard greens, turnip greens, peas, and even avocados all contain these powerful nutrients.

When you're at the farmers' market or browsing the produce aisle at the grocery store, be sure to stock up with a variety of different colors to provide your body with an abundance of different beneficial plant compounds.

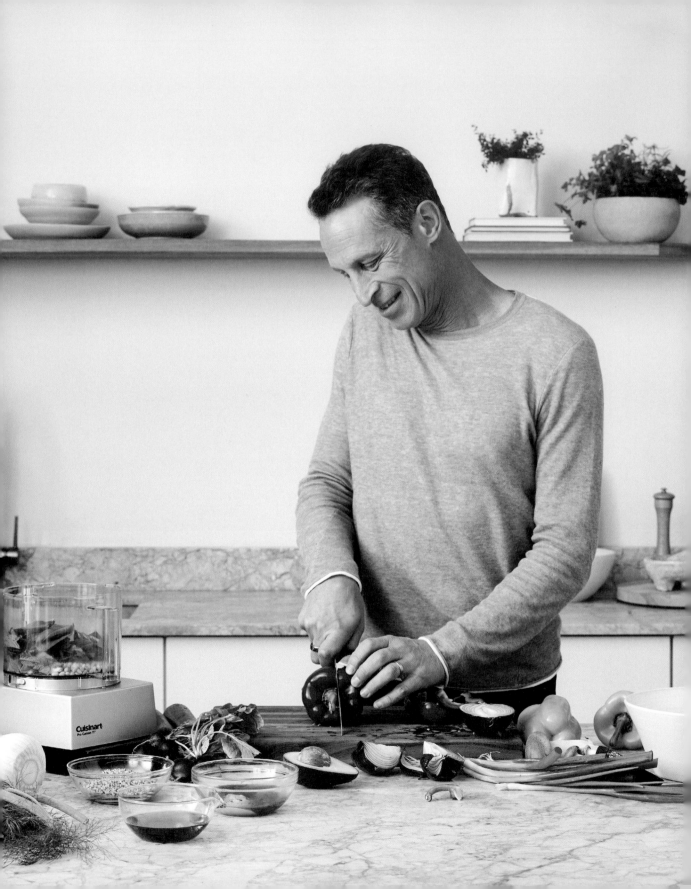

BECOME A CONSCIOUS COOK

My hope is that this book will give you all the tools you need to make your own healthy meals at the drop of a hat. To do that, it's important to be aware of certain cooking principles that can either benefit or destroy the nutritional density of your food. The methods you use matter—meaning you can turn the highest-quality ingredients into a poor-quality meal if you're not a conscious cook.

Cooking with the Right Fats

Certain kinds of seed oils are better to use for drizzling than for cooking, including sesame, flax, and hemp oils; and the same goes for nut oils from almonds, walnuts, and macadamias. These polyunsaturated fats oxidize when exposed to heat and turn into harmful compounds, but when used to season food after cooking they can provide many beneficial nutrients and healthy fats, along with tons of flavor. Extra virgin olive oil also falls into this category.

So, what should you use for cooking? Avocado oil, coconut oil, and ghee are best for high-heat cooking due to their stable saturated fats, which means they have a higher smoke point. And note that if your fats reach their smoke point while you're cooking, beneficial nutrients and phytochemicals will be lost, harmful compounds will be created, and your food will come out with an unpleasant burnt flavor.

Lower and Slower Is Better

High-temperature cooking methods can create carcinogenic by-products and turn what was a high-quality cut of meat into an unhealthy meal. When fats or proteins are exposed to high heat, a chemical reaction takes place resulting in compounds called advanced glycation end products, or AGEs. The name is no coincidence, considering that these harmful toxins accelerate the aging process by increasing oxidative stress and inflammation within the body.[5] The addition of sugar makes this reaction even worse (so avoid those sugary BBQ sauces!).

Change your cooking methods to reduce your exposure to these toxic compounds. Focus on lower-temperature, slow cooking for meat—such as baking, poaching, and stewing—as well as methods that embrace moisture, like cooking in a slow cooker. Using an acidic marinade prior to cooking (think vinegar or lemon juice) can also counteract the negative effects of cooking proteins at high temperatures. Be cautious with your veggies, too—marinating them with anything sugary and cooking at high heat will also produce AGEs.

Soak for Better Digestion

Nuts, seeds, grains, and legumes are all healthy, whole foods, but they can be made more easily digestible by soaking them prior to cooking. That's because soaking them in water mimics the germination process, helps to deactivate certain nutrient inhibitors like phytic acid, releases greater amounts of certain nutrients, and activates enzymes that will assist your body in digesting them. Soaking times vary by ingredient but can easily be found online.

Avoid Boiling

When vegetables are submerged in water and boiled, certain nutrients, like B vitamins and vitamin C, leach into the water. If you toss that water, you toss the nutrients. Blanching, or quickly submerging vegetables in boiling water and then plunging them in an ice bath, can also produce some nutrient loss, though the effects are less than boiling for an extended time. It's better to steam, sauté, or roast vegetables instead. These practices retain more nutrients, plus they incorporate fat that will help your body absorb certain

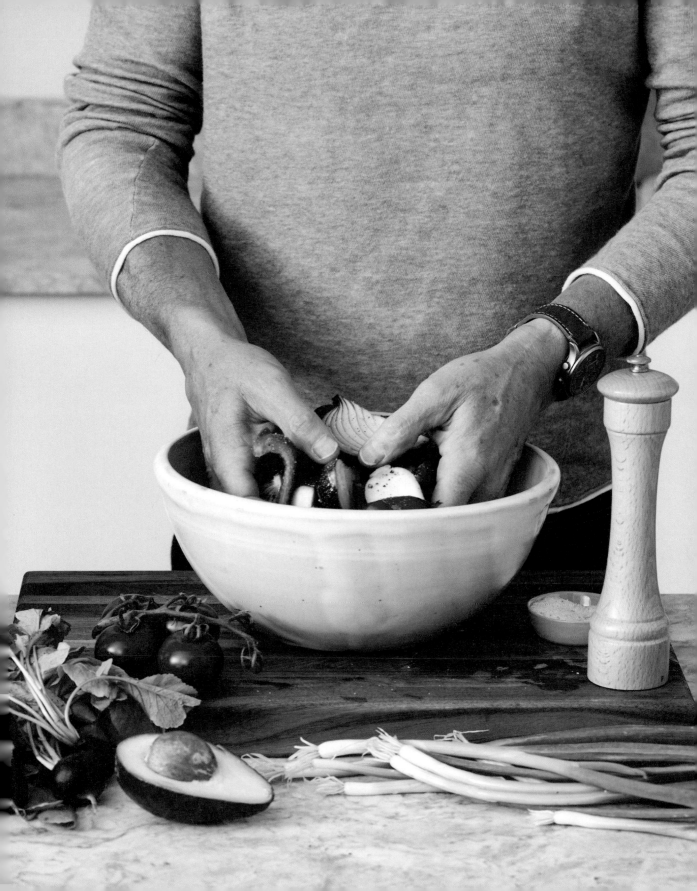

nutrients. Making soups or stews is also a good option because you consume the nutrient-rich liquid the vegetables cook in.

Simple Cooking Techniques for Vegetables

There are lots of hacks to make healthy cooking take less time and energy, and you'll learn about them as you dive into the amazing recipes in this book. To encourage you to experiment with recipe-free cooking and get more comfortable in the kitchen, I'll break down a few of my favorite ways to cook vegetables, since they should be the main part of every single meal.

How to Steam

When you fill up your steamer pot be sure to avoid adding too much water; you don't want the water to touch the veggies and then lose their nutrients in the water. You can steam almost any type of vegetable like this and it takes no time at all:

- Add water to a saucepan fitted with a steamer basket, but be careful that the water doesn't rise up into the basket.

- Bring the water to a boil.

- Place chopped veggies into the steaming basket, cover the pan, and steam for 4 to 8 minutes, depending on the vegetable and your desired level of tenderness.

- Remove the veggies from the basket, add favorite seasonings, and drizzle with some kind of healthy oil, such as extra virgin olive oil, walnut oil, or hemp seed oil.

How to Sauté

Sautéing vegetables is another delicious way to quickly cook a variety of vegetables that can also produce a firmer texture than steaming. However, it's important to use the right fats, as I explained earlier. I prefer to use stable fats like coconut oil, avocado oil, ghee, and grass-fed butter for sautéing my veggies.

- Melt 1 tablespoon of desired oil or butter in a skillet over medium-high heat.

- After several minutes, when the pan is hot and oil is melted or shimmering, add chopped veggies and sprinkle with any desired spices.
- Cook for 5 to 7 minutes, stirring occasionally, until your desired level of tenderness is reached. Sprinkle with sea salt and black pepper to taste.

How to Roast

Though the overall cook time is longer for roasting than it is for steaming and sautéing, it can be a really time-efficient way to prepare vegetables because it's relatively hands-off. That means you can work on another part of the meal like a sauce or dressing, or prepare your lunch or workout bag for the following day, all while dinner is in the works.

- Preheat the oven to 425°F.
- Chop veggies into pieces that are roughly the same size—about ½-inch thick or wide is a good rule of thumb—and place in a mixing bowl.
- Add a suitable fat for high-heat cooking, such as avocado oil, coconut oil, or ghee. Generally speaking, about 1 teaspoon oil is appropriate for every 1 cup of vegetables. Toss to coat the veggies.
- Add your choice of herbs and spices and toss well to coat.
- Spread the veggies on one or two baking sheets. Take care not to crowd them. They should have room to spread out in a single layer, so that moisture can release; this will help you get more of a roasted veggie than a steamed one. It's also helpful to use baking sheets or shallow pans to help the moisture escape more easily.
- Pop your baking sheets in the oven. Give everything a stir after roughly 10 minutes. Continue roasting and checking every 10 minutes, until the veggies are fork-tender. Depending on the vegetables and how small they are cut, they'll need to roast for 20 to 40 minutes.
- Once done, remove from the oven and sprinkle with sea salt and pepper to taste.

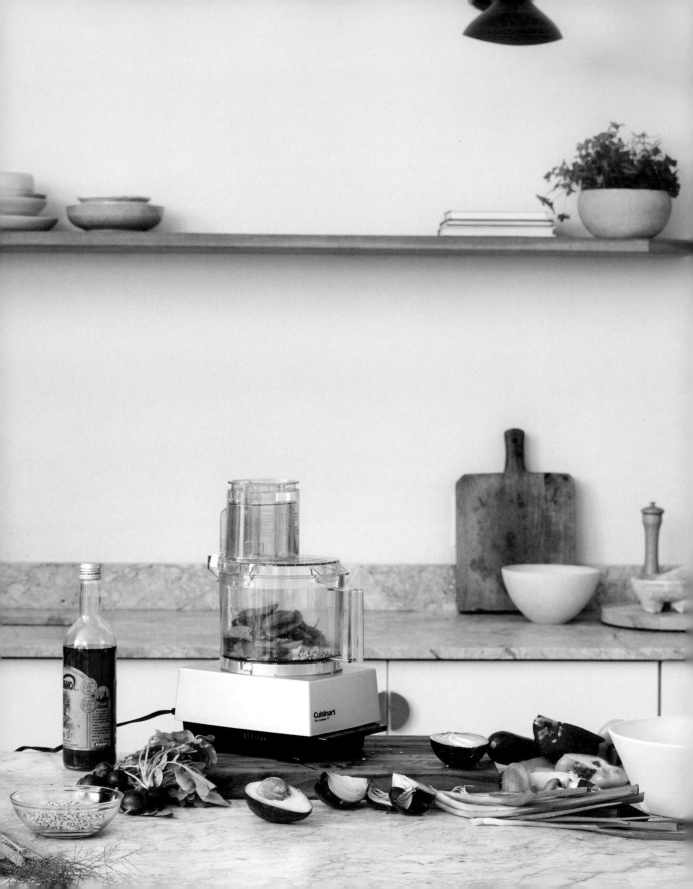

Kitchen Essentials: Gadgets and Tools Every Chef Needs

Simple, healthy food doesn't need a ton of prep work to become a delicious meal. That being said, certain kitchen gadgets can make the job easier and even more fun, plus they can help you get just the right taste and texture. By no means do you need to run out and purchase all of these items to create the recipes in this book, but think of slowly adding to your culinary toolbox as an investment in your health.

Here are my favorite kitchen tools to have around, some of which I'm sure you already have:

Basic Tools

- Good set of knives (keep them sharp, you may also want to purchase a sharpening kit)
- Two or three wooden cutting boards (one for animal foods, one for fruits and vegetables, and some people like to keep a third one for onions and garlic)
- Three glass mixing bowls (small, medium, and large)
- Colander
- Sieve
- Wide, flat silicone spatula for flipping
- Two or three different sizes of silicone spatulas for scraping bowls
- Large wooden or silicone spoons for scooping and mixing

- Measuring cups, metal for dry ingredients and glass for liquids
- Stainless steel measuring spoons
- Garlic press (makes preparing and measuring fresh garlic a breeze)
- Citrus reamer
- Wire whisk
- Spring tongs
- Micro-grater/zester
- Vegetable peeler
- Can opener
- Instant-read thermometer
- Natural parchment paper
- Sealable glass containers in various sizes for storing food

Appliances

- High-speed blender
- Food processor
- Hand mixer
- Large slow cooker/Crockpot or Instant Pot
- Coffee grinder (for nuts, seeds, and spices)
- Spiralizer (for making vegetable noodles)
- Speakers (Just for fun! I like to listen to music while I cook.)

Pots and Pans

- Large and small nonstick, ceramic, stainless steel, or cast-iron sauté pans (be sure the nonstick varieties are nontoxic—look for options that say they're free of PTFE, PFCs, and Teflon)
- Two rimmed baking sheets
- Two silicone baking mats
- Several square and/or rectangular glass or ceramic baking dishes
- Dutch oven
- 8-quart stockpot, with lid
- 2-quart and 4-quart saucepans, with lids
- 11-inch-square nonstick stovetop griddle (be sure it's nontoxic)
- Stovetop grill pan
- Vegetable steaming rack or basket

Are you ready to cook? I hope so! With this book as your guide I have no doubt you'll be creating incredibly delicious, nutritious, Pegan meals for your whole family in no time at all. Remember, this is a lifestyle, not a diet, and every bite is a step toward optimal, long-term health. Now, let's dive into recipes for the first meal of the day—breakfast—with a variety of tasty options to get you started on the right foot.

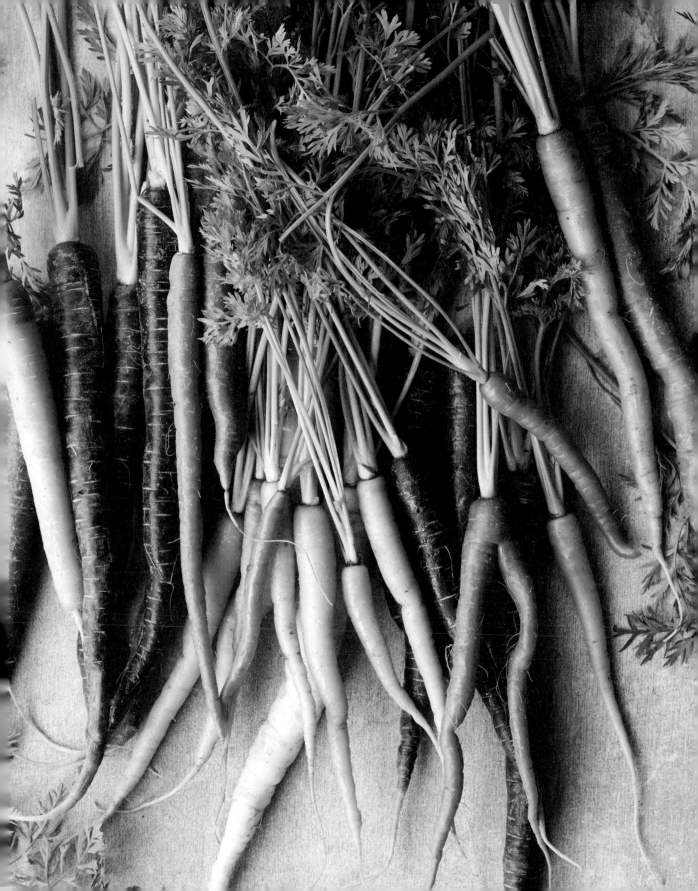

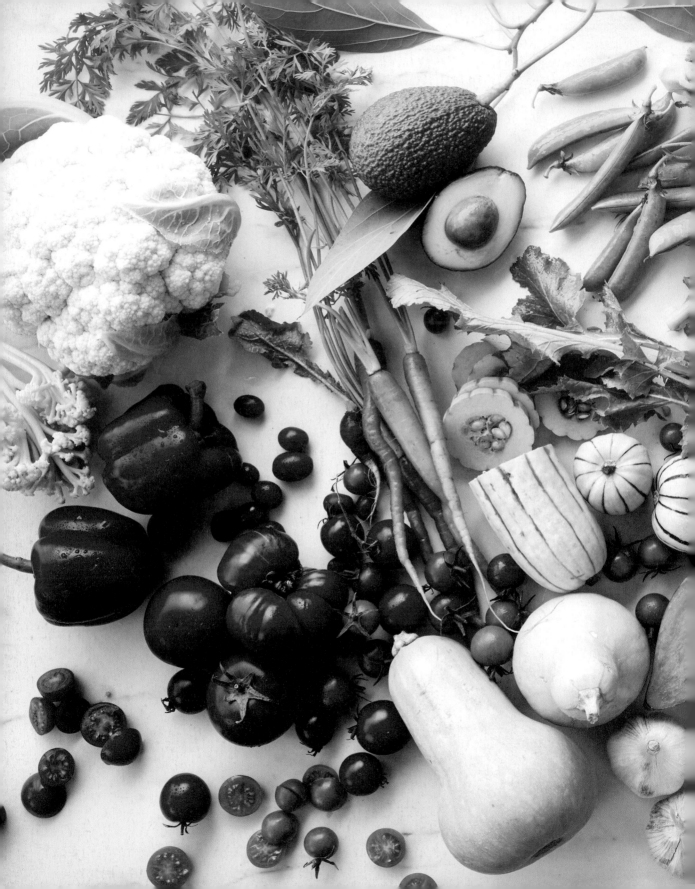

Part III

The Recipes

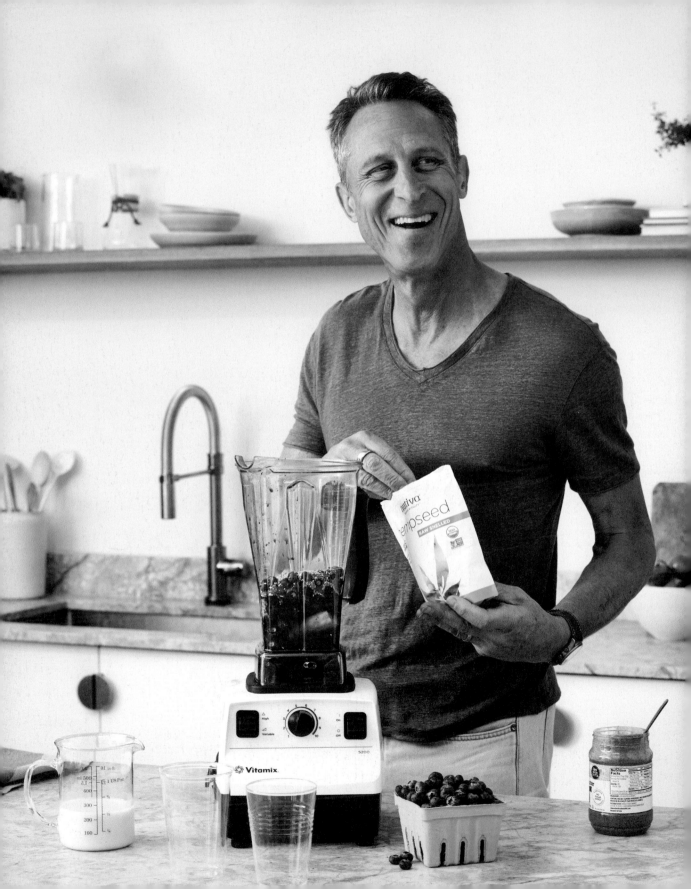

Breakfast

Breakfast is a time to set the stage for a successful day—one built around focus, energy, and conscious choices that elevate your well-being. So many people have grown accustomed to sugary, heavy breakfasts rich in fast-burning carbs, only to find themselves tired, hungry, overweight, and unhappy on a regular basis. Starting the morning with fiber-rich, colorful plant foods, protein, and of course some brain-boosting fat is a game-changer when it comes to how you feel throughout the day. Try all of these mouthwatering recipes to experience the many benefits of a breakfast done right.

Broccoli Breakfast Bowl

Serves: 4

Prep Time: 15 minutes

Cook Time: 10 minutes

Eggs and Broccoli

¾ cup pepitas

8 large pasture-raised eggs

3 heads broccoli, chopped into bite-size pieces (about 6 cups)

3 cups baby arugula, roughly chopped

¼ cup loosely packed fresh cilantro, chopped

Sea salt and freshly ground black pepper, to taste

Dressing

3 tablespoons hemp oil

1 tablespoon gluten-free tamari

1 tablespoon lemon juice

1 teaspoon Dijon mustard

1 teaspoon garlic, pressed

½ teaspoon freshly ground black pepper

Broccoli is probably not the first thing that comes to mind when you think of breakfast, but this recipe is going to change that. Broccoli is a superfood thanks to its diverse nutrient content, plus it contains powerful plant compounds, called sulforaphanes, that are protective against cancer, cardiovascular disease, neurodegeneration, and more. The arugula, pumpkin seeds, eggs, and hemp oil give this breakfast plenty of fiber, protein, and healthy fat—everything you need in one satisfying bowl.

1. Fill one large pot (large enough to hold the eggs without touching) with water and bring to a boil. Add 1 inch water to a second pot and place a steamer basket inside for the broccoli; cover and bring the water to a boil.

2. Heat a medium sauté pan over medium-high heat. Add the pepitas and toast, continuously stirring and shaking the pan, for 4 to 5 minutes, until fragrant and slightly golden. Remove from heat and set aside.

3. Once the water in each pot is boiling, add the eggs to the large pot and the broccoli to the steamer basket in the other pot. Cover the broccoli pot, then boil the eggs and steam the broccoli for 7 minutes, until the broccoli is bright green and tender.

4. Meanwhile, make the dressing: Combine all dressing ingredients in a small bowl and stir well.

5. Drain the eggs and run cold tap water into the pot to stop the cooking process. Allow the eggs to sit in the cold water until cool enough to handle. Rinse the broccoli with cold water, drain well, and transfer to a large bowl.

6. Once the eggs are cool enough to handle, peel and slice each in half.

7. Add the toasted pepitas, arugula, and cilantro to the broccoli and sprinkle with sea salt and pepper to taste. Add the dressing and toss. Divide among four bowls and top with the egg halves.

Eggs and Peppers

CONTRIBUTED BY MEHMET OZ, MD

Serves: 4

Prep Time: 10 minutes
Cook Time: 10 minutes

¼ cup coconut oil

1 large sweet or yellow onion, sliced into rings

1 red bell pepper, stemmed, seeded, and thinly sliced into rings

1 yellow bell pepper, stemmed, seeded, and thinly sliced into rings

1 green bell pepper, stemmed, seeded, and thinly sliced into rings

8 large pasture-raised eggs

2 ripe avocados, pitted, peeled, and sliced

Handful of fresh cilantro, minced

1 small cantaloupe, rind removed, sliced into thin wedges

This delicious recipe comes from my good friend Dr. Mehmet Oz, a leader in the world of wellness who has made amazing efforts to educate Americans about living a healthier life. This simple recipe provides you with beneficial fats from coconut oil and avocado, complete protein from pasture-raised eggs, and nutrients like vitamin C and antioxidants from colorful peppers.

1. Heat the coconut oil in a large skillet over medium-high heat. Add the onion and sauté for 3 to 5 minutes, until golden. Add the peppers and sauté 3 to 5 minutes longer, tossing often, until warm but still crisp. Remove the peppers and onions with tongs, arrange on a plate, and cover with foil to keep warm.

2. Reduce the heat to medium and crack the eggs into the same skillet. Cook the eggs just long enough to firm up the whites while keeping the yolks runny, 2 to 3 minutes. Slide the eggs onto the plate alongside the peppers and onions.

3. To serve, top the eggs with avocado slices arranged in a fan and scatter cilantro on top of the eggs and peppers. Add the cantaloupe wedges on the side.

Buckwheat Blini

1 cup raw buckwheat groats

½ cup plus 2 tablespoons
filtered water

2 tablespoons ground flaxseed

2 teaspoons avocado oil,
plus more for cooking

½ teaspoon baking powder

½ teaspoon sea salt

¼ teaspoon freshly ground
black pepper

1½ teaspoons fresh
thyme leaves

Salmon and Spinach Toppings

1 tablespoon coconut oil
or ghee

3 cloves garlic, pressed
(about 1 tablespoon)

Grated zest of 1 lemon

¼ teaspoon sea salt, plus
more to taste

¼ teaspoon freshly ground
black pepper, plus more to
taste

16 ounces spinach

8 ounces cold, smoked
wild-caught salmon, cut into
16 slices

¼ cup fresh dill, chopped

½ small red onion, thinly sliced

2 lemons, quartered

Buckwheat Blini with Smoked Salmon and Spinach

My buckwheat blini make a delicious base for all sorts of different ingredients. Here, I pair them with smoked wild-caught salmon, spinach, and fresh dill for a savory and unique breakfast that will power up your brain and metabolism for a productive, feel-good day. You can also top them with coconut cream, fruit, and nut butter. Note that you need to soak the buckwheat groats overnight, so plan ahead.

1. Place the buckwheat groats in a medium bowl and add enough water to cover by at least 3 inches. Cover with a lid or clean towel and place in the fridge to soak for at least 8 hours.

2. The next morning, drain the soaked buckwheat groats and rinse well in a sieve.

3. In a blender or food processor, combine the rinsed buckwheat groats, water, flaxseed, avocado oil, baking powder, salt, and pepper and blend until smooth, about 1 minute. Stir the thyme into the batter.

4. Heat a large heavy skillet over medium heat and add about 1 teaspoon avocado oil. Add 2 or 3 portions of batter (about 3 tablespoons each) to the skillet, and use the back of a spoon to spread the batter as thin as possible. Cook the blini until the tops begin to set and the bottoms are lightly browned, about 2 minutes. Flip and cook for another minute, then transfer to a plate. Repeat with more oil and the remaining batter to make 16 blini. Keep the prepared blini warm at low heat in a toaster oven or oven while making the rest.

5. To prepare the toppings: Heat the coconut oil or ghee in a large sauté pan over medium heat, then add the garlic, lemon zest, salt, and pepper. Cook and stir well until fragrant, about 1 minute. In small batches, add the spinach to the pan and continuously mix so the cold spinach is mixed into the warm spinach. It should take about 10 minutes for it all to cook down. Add salt and pepper to taste once thoroughly cooked. Drain the spinach in a colander, using tongs to help squeeze out water.

6. Top each blini with warm spinach, 1 slice smoked salmon, a pinch of dill, and a few slices of red onion and serve with lemon wedges on the side.

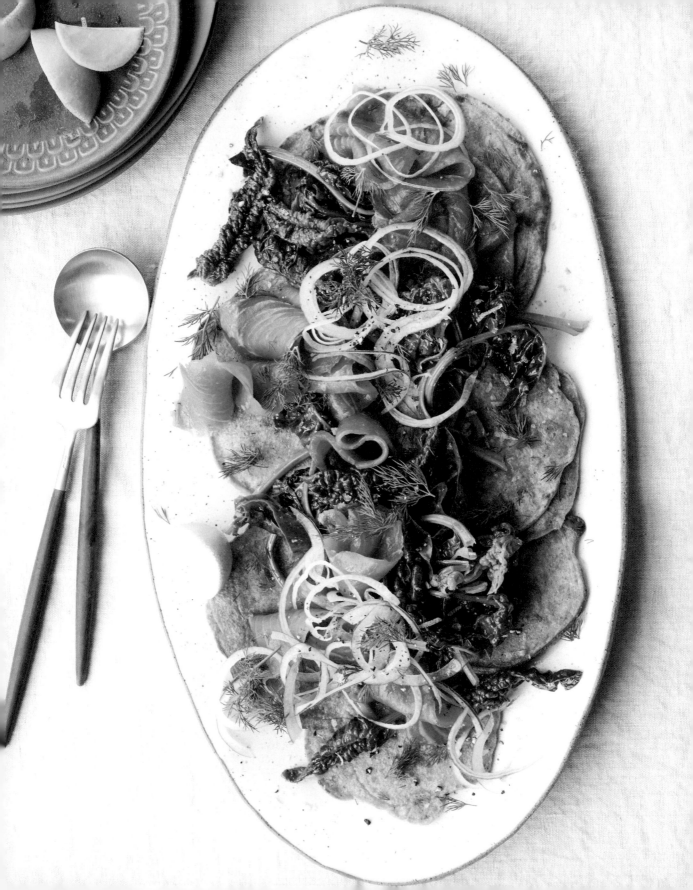

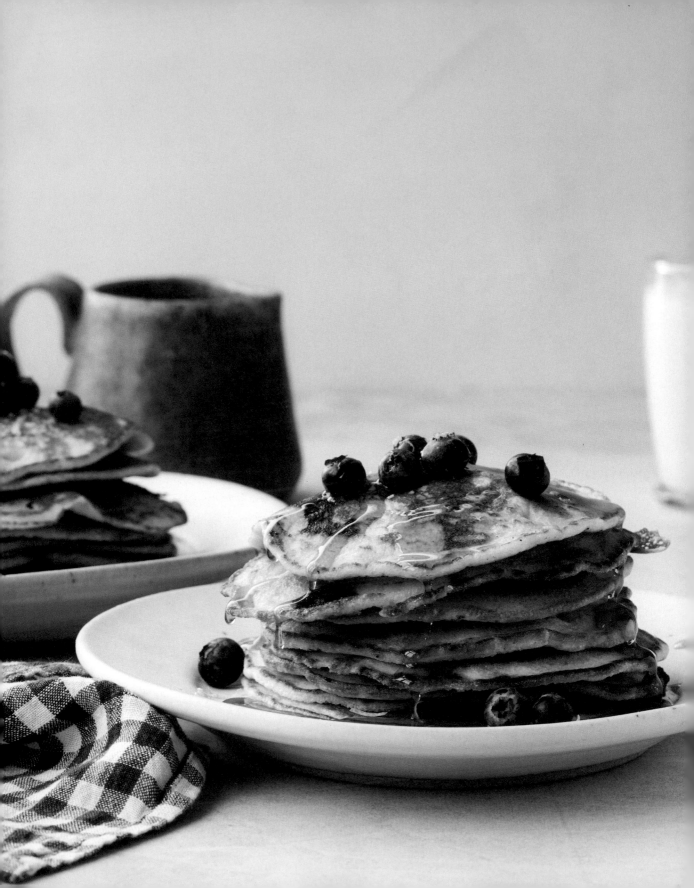

Grain-Free Lemon-Blueberry Pancakes

Makes: 12 (4-inch)
pancakes

Prep Time: 10 minutes
Cook Time: 40 minutes

6 large pasture-raised eggs

1½ cups light unsweetened coconut milk

3 tablespoons lemon juice

1½ tablespoons raw honey (optional)

1 tablespoon vanilla extract

¾ cup cassava flour

¾ teaspoon baking powder

Pinch of sea salt

¼ cup plus 2 tablespoons coconut flour

1½ tablespoons grated lemon zest, plus more for garnish

About 6 teaspoons coconut oil

1¼ cups fresh blueberries

Maple syrup (optional)

These pancakes will make you forget all about the refined-flour, sugar-laden ones of your childhood. Lemon zest and fresh blueberries give them a bright, fresh flavor and coconut flour contributes lots of fiber, so they're extremely satisfying. Eggs provide a nice amount of protein and B vitamins to help start your day.

1. In a large bowl, whisk together the eggs, coconut milk, lemon juice, honey (if using), and vanilla until well combined. Mix in the cassava flour, baking powder, and sea salt, then use a sieve to sift in the coconut flour and stir well. Fold in the lemon zest and let the batter rest for 3 minutes.

2. Heat 1 teaspoon coconut oil in a large skillet over medium heat. When the pan is hot and the oil is melted, add two portions of batter (¼ cup each) to the pan and immediately sprinkle a small handful of blueberries on the top of each. Cook for 3 minutes, then flip the pancakes and cook for another 3 to 4 minutes, until golden brown. Use a spatula to transfer pancakes to a plate and cover with foil to keep warm.

3. Repeat with the remaining batter and oil as needed to make 12 pancakes.

4. To serve, top the pancakes with the remaining blueberries, additional lemon zest, and a little drizzle of maple syrup if desired.

Green Shakshuka

Serves: 4

Prep Time: 10 minutes
Cook Time: 20 to
25 minutes

2 tablespoons coconut oil

2 large leeks, thinly sliced

1 bunch kale, chopped

2 large cloves garlic, minced

1 teaspoon caraway seeds

½ teaspoon sea salt

¼ teaspoon chili flakes

¾ cup full-fat unsweetened
coconut milk (half of a
13.5-ounce can)

4 large pasture-raised eggs

Shakshuka, a popular Israeli breakfast of eggs cooked in a flavorful sauce, is a delicious meal any time of day. It's often made with a tomato-based sauce, but this variation features poached eggs in a saucy, green blend of leeks, kale, and coconut milk. Rich in protein, fiber, and healthy fats, this savory meal will easily work its way into your weekly rotation.

1. Preheat the oven to 350°F.

2. In a 10-inch ovenproof skillet, warm the coconut oil over medium-high heat until shimmering. Add the leeks and cook, stirring occasionally, until soft, about 3 minutes. Stir in the kale and continue to cook for another 2 minutes. Stir in the garlic, caraway seeds, salt, and chili flakes and cook until fragrant, about 3 minutes.

3. Add the coconut milk and bring to a simmer. Carefully crack each egg into the green sauce, spacing evenly. Transfer the pan to the oven and bake for 10 to 12 minutes, until the egg whites solidify and the yolks are cooked to desired doneness. Serve immediately.

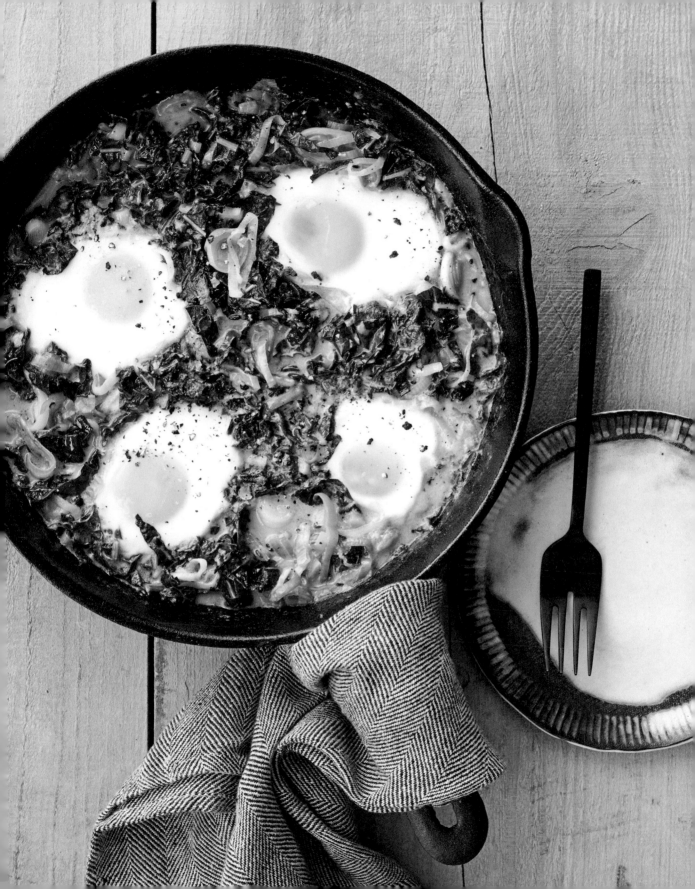

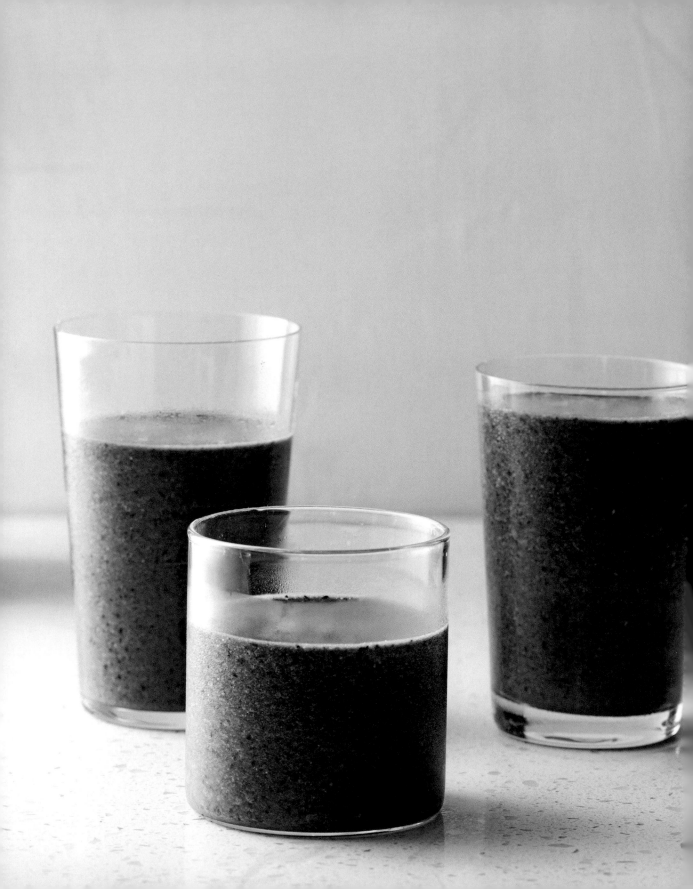

Morning Glory
Collagen Smoothie

Serves: 1

Prep Time: 5 minutes

½ cup wild blueberries

½ small zucchini, peeled and frozen

2 scoops (about 2 tablespoons) collagen powder

½ cup almond milk

½ cup coconut water

1 tablespoon almond butter

1 teaspoon chia seeds

1 teaspoon hemp seeds

1 teaspoon MCT oil or coconut oil

¼ teaspoon ground cinnamon

A rich and creamy smoothie is a delicious way to start the day. Wild blueberries are one of the best sources of antioxidants on the planet, plus they've been found to support memory, cognitive function, and mood. The collagen powder provides protein while the almond butter, chia seeds, hemp seeds, and MCT oil all provide healthy fats that will fill you up, help you absorb key nutrients, and keep you energized throughout the morning. To plan ahead, wash, chop, and freeze your zucchini the night before.

1. Combine all ingredients in a blender and blend until smooth. Pour into a glass and enjoy.

Orange-Blackberry Almond Scones

Makes: 6 scones

Prep Time: 15 minutes
Cook Time: 18 to
20 minutes

2 cups almond flour

½ cup millet flour

2 tablespoons coconut sugar
(optional)

1 teaspoon baking powder

½ teaspoon ground cinnamon

¼ teaspoon sea salt

2 tablespoons coconut oil,
melted but not hot

2 large pasture-raised eggs

1½ teaspoons vanilla extract

Grated zest of 3 oranges

¾ cup blackberries

Blackberries are one of my absolute favorite fruits—they're a great source of vitamin C and contain many other antioxidants that are protective against inflammation, cancer, neurological diseases, and more. Thanks to almond and millet flours, these scones are a nutrient-dense, lower-glycemic alternative to traditional scones that are made with refined flour and sugar, plus they provide healthy fats and protein to keep you satiated.

1. Preheat the oven to 375°F and line a baking sheet with parchment paper.

2. In a medium bowl, combine the almond flour, millet flour, coconut sugar (if using), baking powder, cinnamon, and salt. In another medium bowl, combine the coconut oil, eggs, vanilla, and orange zest. Stir well. Add the egg mixture to the almond flour mixture, stirring well. Gently fold the blackberries into the dough.

3. Lay a square piece of parchment paper on the counter. Place the dough on the parchment and flatten into a 1-inch-thick disk. Cut the disk in half, then slice each half into 3 wedges, creating 6 pieces. Place the scones on the lined baking sheet and bake for 18 to 20 minutes, until golden brown.

4. Let cool for a few minutes before serving. Store leftover scones in an airtight container in the fridge for up to 2 days.

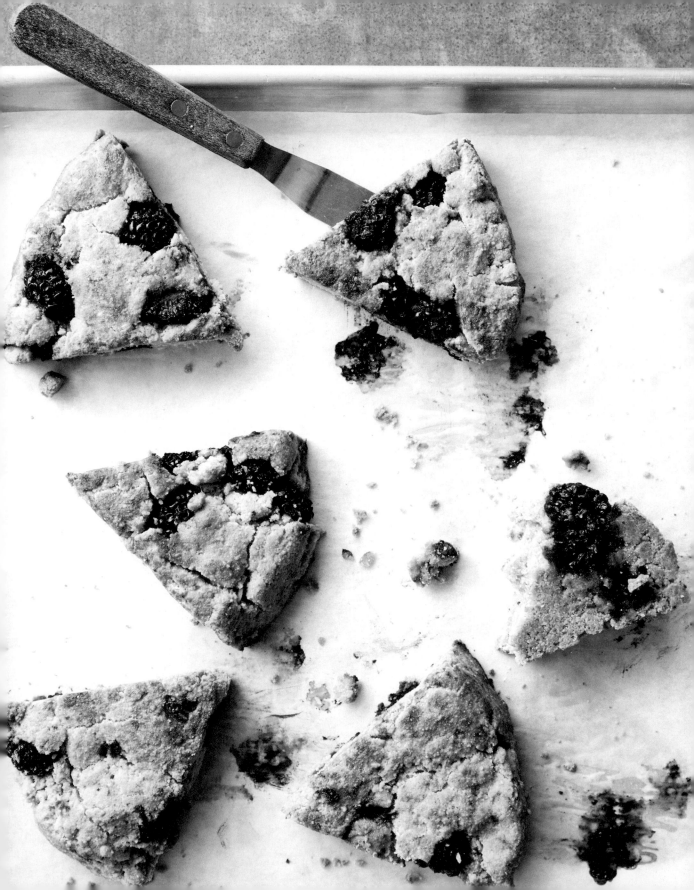

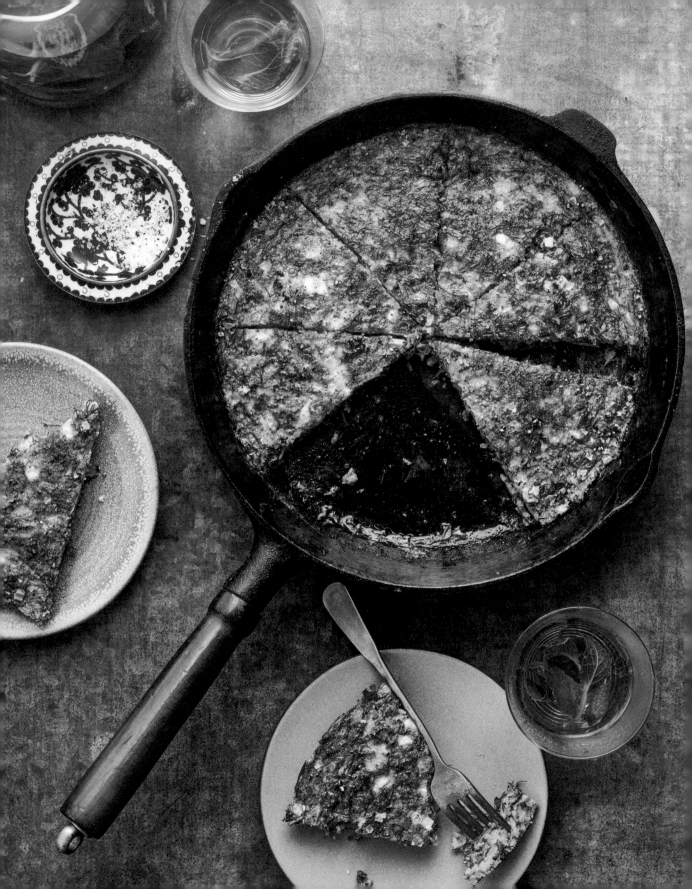

Persian Green-Herb Omelet

Serves: 4

Prep Time: 10 minutes
Cook Time: 10 minutes

6 large pasture-raised eggs

½ cup finely chopped
green onions

½ cup loosely packed fresh
parsley leaves, finely chopped

½ cup loosely packed fresh
cilantro leaves, finely chopped

½ cup loosely packed fresh dill,
finely chopped

¼ teaspoon ground cumin

¼ teaspoon ground turmeric

1 teaspoon sea salt

½ teaspoon black pepper

1 tablespoon avocado oil
or ghee

1 small white onion, finely
grated

This savory omelet is packed with protein and fresh, fragrant herbs. I love the addition of turmeric for its potent anti-inflammatory effects, which are made more bioavailable when combined with black pepper and the healthy fats found in avocado oil. This recipe sounds fancy, but it's easy to make and goes great with a bed of mixed greens tossed with olive oil.

1. Beat the eggs in a large bowl and add the green onions, parsley, cilantro, dill, cumin, turmeric, salt, and pepper.

2. Warm the avocado oil or ghee in a cast-iron skillet over medium heat until shimmering. Add the grated onion and cook until translucent. Add the egg mixture and combine well with the onions. Increase the heat to high and cook for 1 minute without stirring. Turn the heat to low, cover the skillet, and cook for 4 to 6 minutes, until the mixture is no longer runny but not completely set.

3. Turn the broiler to high. Uncover the skillet, place on the top shelf of the oven, and broil just until eggs are set and golden brown, 1 to 2 minutes, depending on your oven.

4. To serve, cut the omelet into triangular slices and use a spatula to plate.

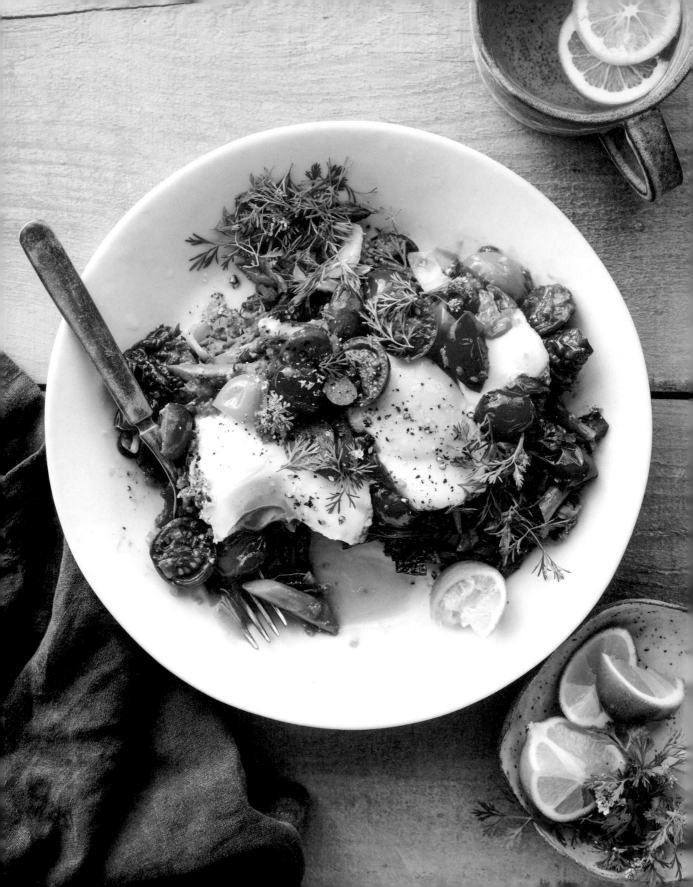

Poached-Egg Power Bowl

I love eggs. They are bursting with complete protein, vitamins, and minerals and it's been shown that eating them in the morning reduces your appetite throughout the rest of the day. Poaching eggs in a vibrant bell pepper and tomato salsa makes them extremely flavorful and provides a much-needed change from that scrambled-egg rut so many of us fall into. Serving it all over sautéed sweet potatoes, bok choy, asparagus, and spinach makes a breakfast bowl with a wide variety of nutrients that will surely power you up and leave you feeling your best.

Serves: 4

Prep Time: 15 minutes
Cook Time: 40 to
45 minutes

Veggies

1 tablespoon avocado oil

1 medium sweet potato, peeled and grated (about 2 cups)

3 cloves garlic, pressed

1 teaspoon ground cumin

½ teaspoon sea salt

2 cups chopped asparagus

1½ cups thinly sliced baby bok choy

3 cups spinach

Eggs and Salsa

2 teaspoons avocado oil

1 small red bell pepper, cored, seeded, and chopped (about 1 cup)

3 medium jalapeños, seeded and minced (about ½ cup), optional

1 medium red onion, minced (about 1 cup)

1 teaspoon sea salt

Freshly ground black pepper

2 pints cherry tomatoes, halved (about 4 cups)

½ teaspoon ground cumin

8 large pasture-raised eggs

Garnish

1 cup loosely packed fresh cilantro leaves, minced

1 lime, quartered

1. Start with the veggies: Warm the avocado oil in a large sauté pan over medium heat until shimmering. Add the sweet potato, garlic, cumin, and salt and cook for about 5 minutes, until the sweet potato is cooked through. Add the asparagus and sauté 5 minutes, then add the baby bok choy and continue cooking another 5 minutes, until the asparagus is just fork tender and the bok choy has wilted. Turn the heat to low and add the spinach, stirring well. Keep the veggies on low heat, stirring occasionally, while you make the eggs and salsa.

2. For the eggs and salsa: Warm the avocado oil in another large sauté pan over medium heat. Add the bell pepper, jalapeño (if using), onion, and ½ teaspoon of the salt and cook until the vegetables begin to soften, about 8 minutes. Add a sprinkle of freshly ground pepper.

3. Add the tomatoes, cumin, and remaining ½ teaspoon salt and continue to cook for another 12 minutes, until the onions and tomatoes are cooked through and the salsa has cooked down. Spread the salsa equally around the pan and reduce the heat to low.

4. Crack each egg into the salsa, spacing evenly. Cover the pan with a lid and cook over low heat for 5 to 7 minutes, depending on preferred doneness for the eggs.

5. To serve, divide the veggies among four bowls. Top each bowl with two eggs and some of the salsa. Garnish each with ¼ cup cilantro and a lime wedge. Serve warm.

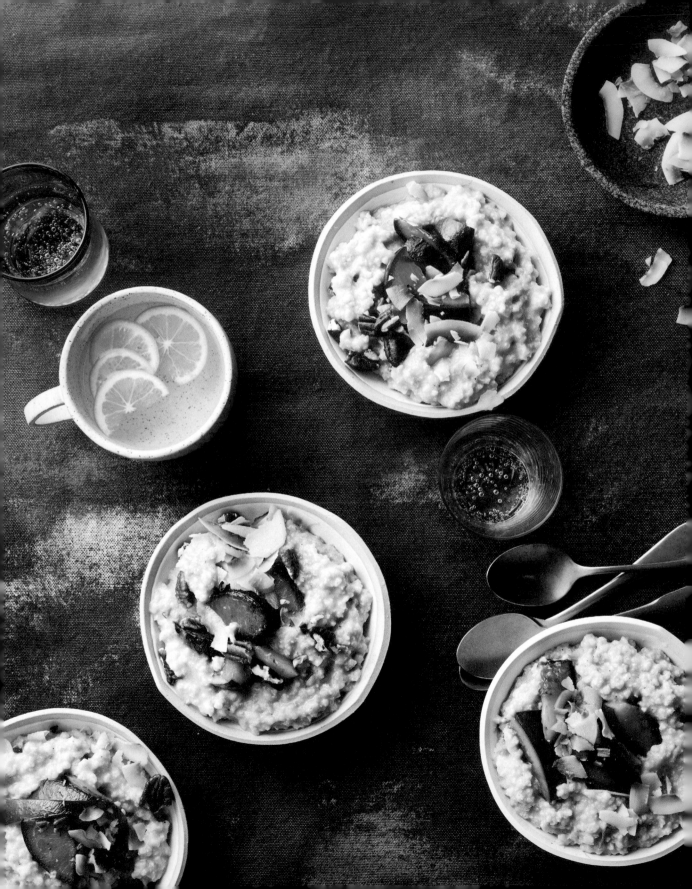

Millet Porridge with Roasted Stone Fruit

Serves: 6

Prep Time: 10 minutes

Cook Time: 25 minutes

Roasted Stone Fruit

3 large plums (or any seasonal stone fruit, such as peaches or nectarines), pitted and quartered

2 teaspoons coconut oil or ghee

Pinch of ground cinnamon

2 teaspoons maple syrup (optional)

Porridge

¾ cup millet

½ cup toasted unsweetened shredded coconut

2 cups light unsweetened coconut milk (or almond milk)

3 cups filtered water

4 scoops (about ¼ cup) collagen powder

½ teaspoon vanilla extract

¼ teaspoon grated nutmeg

½ teaspoon ground cardamom

1 teaspoon ground cinnamon

Pinch of sea salt

Toppings

½ cup toasted unsweetened flaked coconut

½ cup raw pecans, chopped

Sometimes you just want a warm, comforting breakfast—this is the perfect recipe for those cold mornings when you're craving a toasty, satisfying start to the day. Cinnamon, nutmeg, and cardamom add just the right amount of spice to the thick porridge, and you can use any stone fruit. A few scoops of collagen powder provide a boost of protein and healing benefits for the skin and gut.

1. To roast the fruit: Heat the oven to 425°F. Toss the plums with the coconut oil, cinnamon, and maple syrup (if using) and place in a small pan or baking dish. Roast for 5 minutes, then flip and roast another 5 minutes, until the fruit is caramelized. Chop into bite-size pieces.

2. For the porridge: While the fruit is roasting, grind the millet in a high-speed blender until crushed, but avoid blending into a fine flour.

3. In a medium saucepan, whisk together the ground millet, coconut, 1 cup of the coconut milk, water, collagen powder, vanilla, nutmeg, cardamom, cinnamon, and salt. Bring the mixture to a boil, stirring often. Reduce the heat to low and simmer until the millet is soft, 15 to 18 minutes. Add a splash more water if it becomes too thick to easily stir.

4. Divide the porridge among six bowls. Top each with the roasted fruit and garnish with toasted coconut and pecans. Serve with the remaining 1 cup coconut milk.

5. Leftover porridge can be refrigerated for up to 3 days; reheat with a splash of coconut milk when you're ready to enjoy, then add toppings.

Strawberry-Vanilla Chia Pudding

Serves: 1

Prep Time: 10 minutes
Cook Time: 5 to 7 minutes
Chill Time: 4 hours or overnight

2 tablespoons macadamia nuts

1 cup fresh strawberries, chopped

¾ cup canned light unsweetened coconut milk

1 scoop (about 1 tablespoon) collagen powder

2 tablespoons chia seeds

1 teaspoon raw honey (optional)

1 teaspoon vanilla extract

¼ teaspoon ground cinnamon

1 tablespoon unsweetened shredded coconut

Pinch of sea salt

Grated zest of ½ lemon

Here's an easy breakfast to prepare the night before, so you can grab it on your way out the door on a busy morning. Chia seeds are abundant in omega-3 fatty acids and fiber while strawberries provide lots of vitamin C and antioxidants. Collagen powder is a great way to add extra protein to any recipe, and it helps repair connective tissue, support the immune system, and enhance nutrient absorption, among other benefits.

1. Preheat the oven to 350°F. Place macadamia nuts on an ungreased baking sheet and toast for 5 to 7 minutes, until fragrant and slightly golden.

2. Combine ¾ cup of the strawberries, the coconut milk, collagen powder, chia seeds, honey (if using), vanilla, and cinnamon in a small food processor and blend until smooth. Cover the pudding and refrigerate for at least 4 hours or overnight to set.

3. Combine the toasted macadamia nuts, shredded coconut, and sea salt in a small food processor and pulse a few times, until crumbly.

4. Garnish servings of the chia pudding with the remaining ¼ cup chopped strawberries, the macadamia crumble, and lemon zest.

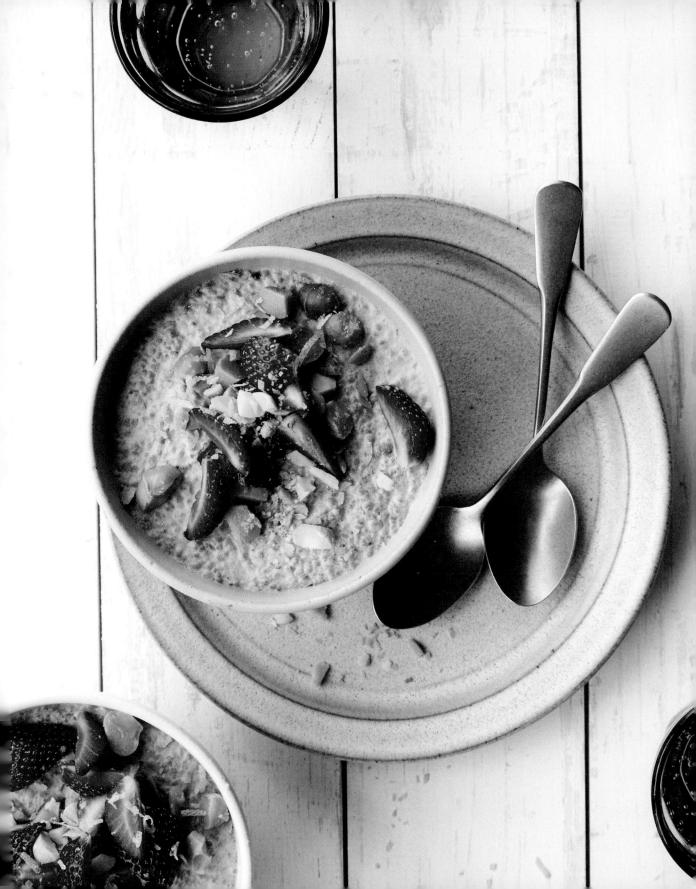

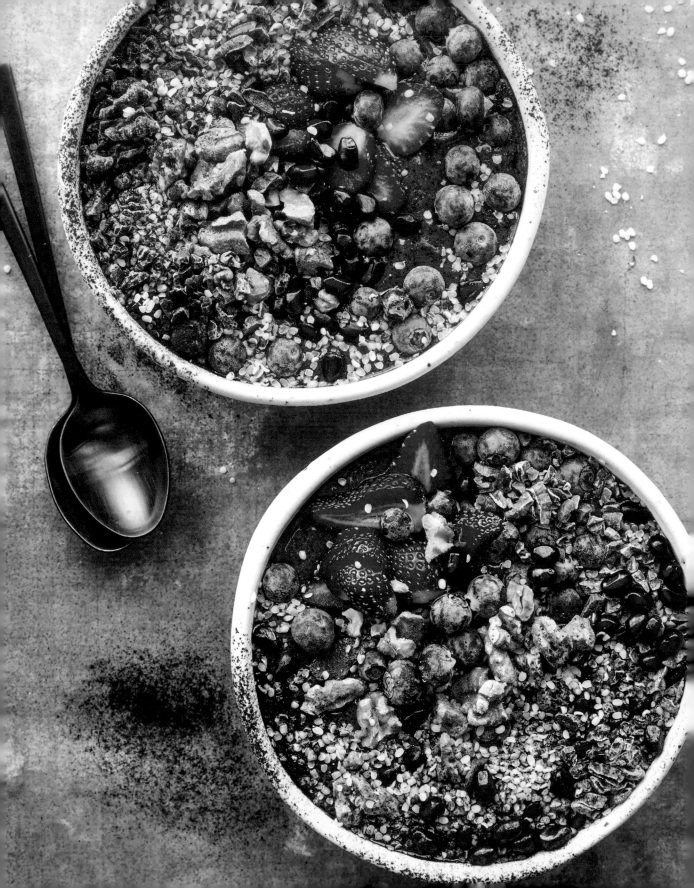

Superfood Smoothie Bowl

Smoothies aren't just for drinking. This smoothie *bowl* lets you enjoy a thicker consistency with an ever-so-satisfying crunch on top. The MCT oil provides energy-boosting fats while the fresh ginger fights dangerous inflammation. Blueberries and spinach are two of my favorite brain-boosting foods, thanks to their respective amounts of anthocyanins and vitamin K—together, they elevate this smoothie bowl to another level.

Serves: 1

Prep Time: 5 minutes
Cook Time: 8 minutes

Spiced Walnuts

¼ cup raw walnuts, chopped and toasted

¼ teaspoon ground cinnamon

Pinch of sea salt

Smoothie Base

1 cup loosely packed baby spinach

½ cup frozen blueberries

¼ cup frozen cauliflower

½ cup filtered water

1 tablespoon MCT oil

1 tablespoon almond butter

1 teaspoon lemon juice

1 teaspoon vanilla extract

1 teaspoon spirulina powder, plus more for garnish

1 teaspoon micro-grated peeled fresh ginger

¼ teaspoon ground cinnamon

Toppings

¼ cup fresh blueberries

¼ cup chopped fresh strawberries

2 teaspoons pomegranate seeds

1½ teaspoons cacao nibs

1 teaspoon hemp seeds

1. For the walnuts: Preheat the oven to 350°F. Place the walnuts on a baking sheet and toast for 8 minutes, until fragrant. In a small bowl, combine the walnuts with the cinnamon and salt. Toss to coat, then set aside to cool.

2. For the smoothie base: Combine all the ingredients in a high-speed blender and purée until smooth.

3. For the toppings: Pour the smoothie into a bowl and garnish with the spiced walnuts, blueberries, strawberries, pomegranate seeds, cacao nibs, and hemp seeds. Sprinkle a dusting of spirulina on top and enjoy.

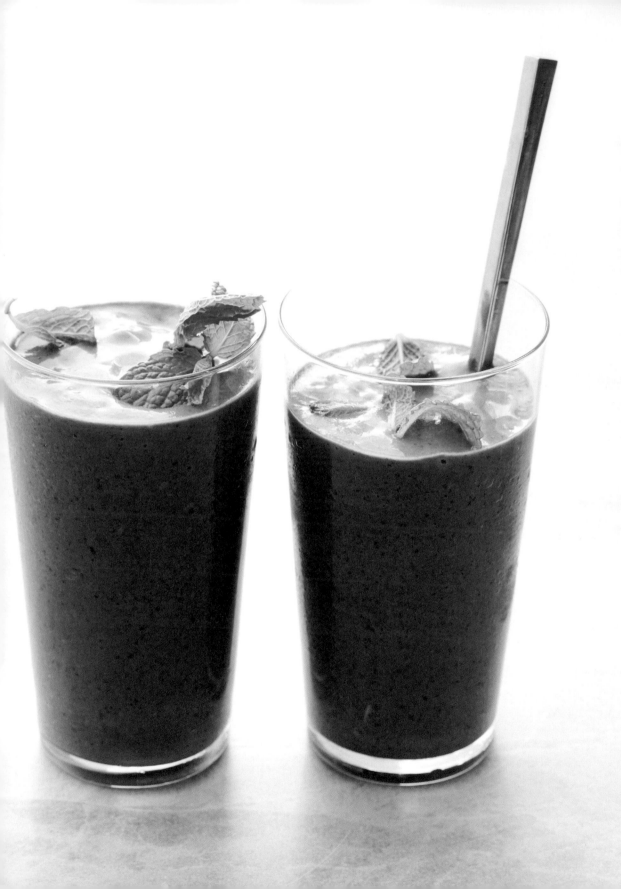

Ultimate Mint Chocolate Shake

Featuring fragrant fresh mint and creamy avocado, this chocolate treat will fill you up and leave you feeling focused and happy. Chocolate can actually be a very healthy part of your breakfast. Cacao powder is incredibly rich in antioxidants, magnesium, and mood-boosting phytochemicals. It also has energizing properties to help you power up for a big day.

Serves: 1

Prep Time: 5 minutes

2 cups unsweetened vanilla almond milk

⅓ cup tightly packed fresh mint leaves, chopped, plus more for garnish

½ large avocado, pitted and peeled

1 to 2 scoops (1 to 2 tablespoons) collagen powder

1½ tablespoons raw cacao powder

1 Medjool date, chopped (optional)

2 ice cubes

Pinch of sea salt

1. Combine all ingredients in a high-speed blender and blend on high until smooth and creamy. Serve with a sprig of fresh mint.

Zucchini Latkes with Lemon-Basil Guacamole

Makes: 18 to 22 latkes
(about 6 servings)

Prep Time: 35 minutes, plus
20 minutes standing
Cook Time: 45 minutes

Lemon-Basil Guacamole

1½ medium avocados, pitted, peeled, and coarsely chopped

3 tablespoons minced green onions

2 tablespoons capers, minced

1 tablespoon finely chopped fresh basil

Grated zest of 1 lemon

2 teaspoons gluten-free tamari

¼ teaspoon freshly ground black pepper

Zucchini Latkes

8 medium zucchini, unpeeled, grated on largest side of a box grater (about 9 cups)

1 tablespoon sea salt

1½ cups almond flour

4 large pasture-raised eggs, beaten

1½ cups baby spinach, finely chopped

½ cup tightly packed fresh basil, finely chopped

½ cup grated red onion

½ cup finely chopped green onions

1 tablespoon garlic powder

These delicious zucchini pancakes are an amazing way to start the day—or end it, for that matter. Combined with eggs, almond flour, fresh spinach, and lots of herbs, grated zucchini is the perfect fiber-rich base for the savory pancakes, which are also a great source of vitamin K, potassium, and folate. Top them with my zesty Lemon-Basil Guacamole for another nutritious layer of flavor and texture.

1. For the guacamole: In a medium bowl, mash together all the ingredients with a fork. Set aside.

2. For the latkes: In a large bowl, combine the grated zucchini and salt. Massage the mixture together until the salt is evenly distributed. Let the mixture sit and drain in a colander for 20 minutes while the zucchini releases excess moisture. Gently squeeze the zucchini over the sink to remove extra water. Once squeezed, you'll end up with about 7 cups total.

3. In a large bowl, combine the zucchini with the almond flour, eggs, spinach, basil, red onion, green onions, garlic powder, paprika, chili powder, baking powder, salt, and pepper. Stir until combined.

4. Warm ½ teaspoon of the coconut oil or ghee in a large skillet over medium heat, until shimmering. Add two portions of batter (about ¼ cup each) to the hot skillet. Cook the latkes until the bottoms are browned and the tops have set, about 2 minutes. If the bottoms appear to darken too quickly, turn the heat down. Flip and cook the other sides for another 2 minutes, then use a spatula to transfer to a paper towel–lined plate. Cover with foil to keep warm.

5. Cook the remaining batter in the same manner to make about 20 latkes, using about ½ teaspoon coconut oil or ghee for every two latkes. Use up the batter as quickly as possible so the zucchini does not continue to release water.

6. Serve the warm latkes with dollops of guacamole.

½ teaspoon smoked paprika

¼ teaspoon chili powder

1 teaspoon baking powder

½ teaspoon sea salt

½ teaspoon freshly ground black pepper

About 2 tablespoons coconut oil or ghee

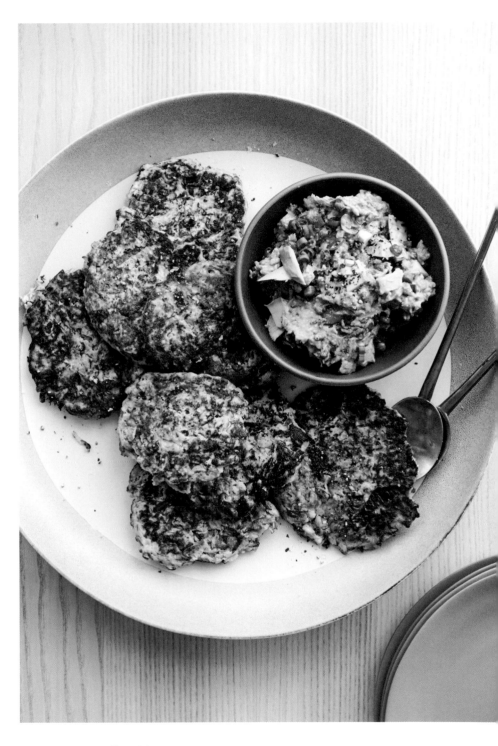

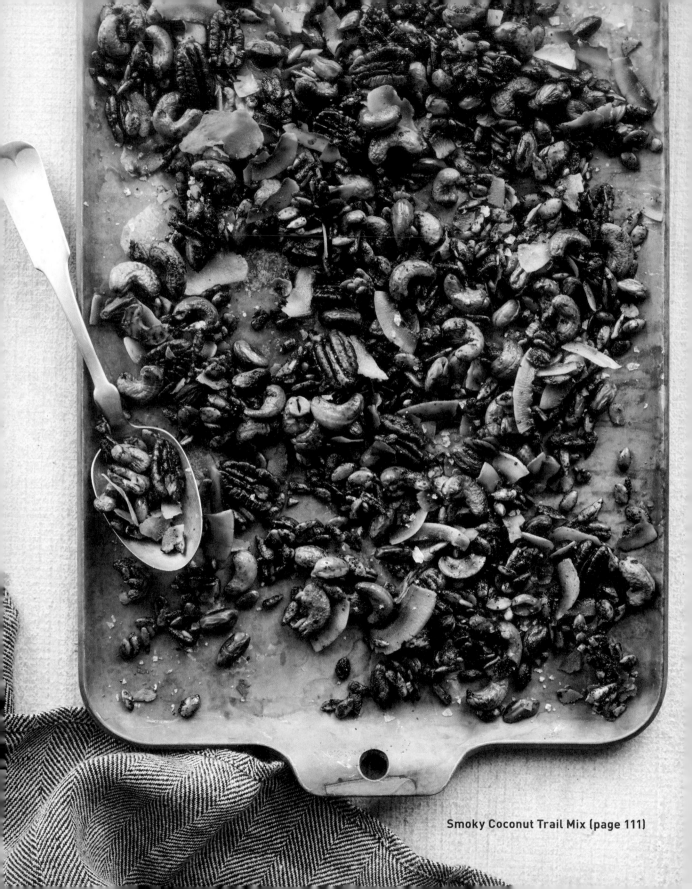

Smoky Coconut Trail Mix (page 111)

Snacks

Sometimes you just need a snack. One meal has come and gone, the next is a couple hours away—but your body is craving an energy boost. This is a moment that can make or break your dietary goals. Reaching for the right foods to snack on, real ones that provide sustainable energy, is an essential part of healthy eating. The recipes in this section are meant to give you the push you need while being satiating in small amounts, thanks to plenty of nutrient-dense ingredients. Take a little time on the weekends to prepare healthy snacks like these and you'll feel great all week long.

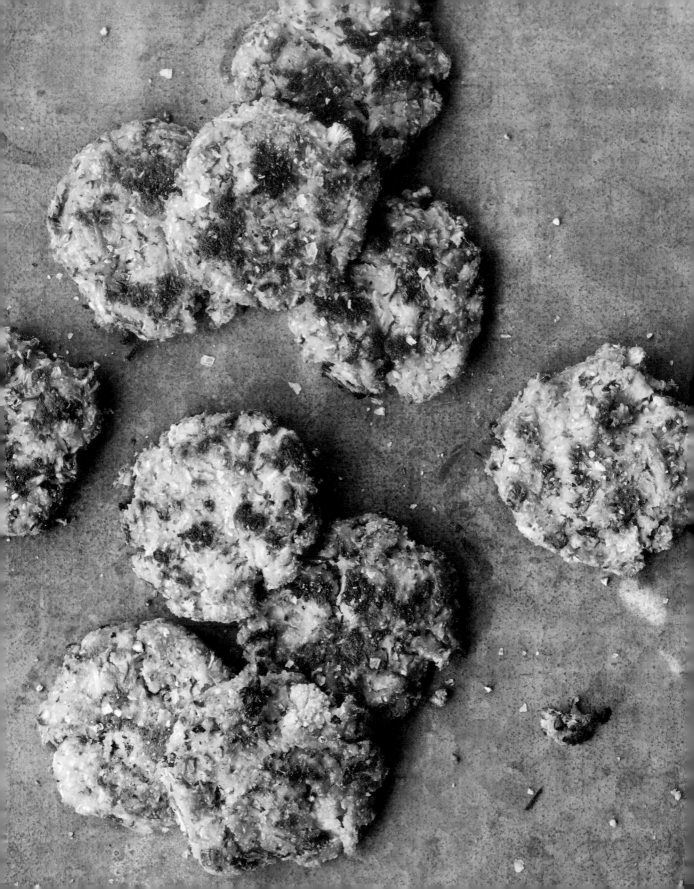

Almond Cauliflower Fritters

Makes: 25 fritters

Prep Time: 20 minutes, plus
15 minutes standing

Cook Time: 35 minutes

2 teaspoons avocado oil

2 medium zucchini, unpeeled,
grated (about 4 cups)

1 teaspoon sea salt

1 medium cauliflower, grated
(about 6 cups)

½ cup fresh cilantro,
finely chopped

½ cup grated white onion

¼ cup finely chopped
green onions

2 teaspoons micro-grated
peeled fresh ginger

2 teaspoons gluten-free tamari

2 teaspoons onion powder

1½ teaspoons garlic powder

1 teaspoon smoked paprika

½ teaspoon ground cumin

½ teaspoon freshly ground
black pepper

1 cup almond flour

These tasty fritters are an easy way to get more veggies into your
day, and they're especially great for kids. They have lots of fiber,
vitamin C, folate from the zucchini and cauliflower, and vitamin E
from the almond flour, which promotes healthy skin and a strong
immune system. Enjoy them hot or cold, and try dipping them in my
Tangy Tomato Basil Sauce (page 275).

1. Preheat the oven to 400°F. Line two baking sheets with parchment
   paper and grease the paper with the avocado oil; set the pans aside.

2. In a colander, toss the grated zucchini with ½ teaspoon of the salt and
   drain in the sink for 15 minutes. Squeeze the grated zucchini to remove
   any excess moisture so it is as dry as possible.

3. In a large bowl, combine the cauliflower, cilantro, white onion, green
   onions, ginger, tamari, onion powder, garlic powder, paprika, cumin,
   remaining ½ teaspoon salt, and black pepper. Add the drained zucchini
   and stir to combine. Add the almond flour and mix well.

4. Scoop 2 tablespoons of the mixture into the palm of your hand and
   shape into a small patty. Repeat to make 25 patties, placing them on the
   two prepared baking sheets. Bake for 15 minutes. Gently flip the
   patties, rotate the pans between oven racks, and bake for another 15 to
   20 minutes, until the fritters are golden. Enjoy the fritters warm or
   cold. They will keep in the fridge for up to 4 days.

Crazy Sexy Trail Mix

CONTRIBUTED BY KRIS CARR

Makes: 2 cups

Prep Time: 5 minutes

½ cup raw Brazil nuts

½ cup raw walnuts

⅓ cup raw cashews

⅓ cup raisins

⅓ cup dried goji berries

2 tablespoons flaked or shredded unsweetened coconut

1 teaspoon ground cinnamon (optional)

I always say real, healthy food doesn't have to be hard to make. This recipe from my friend Kris Carr, a best-selling author, wellness advocate, and cancer thriver, is a great example of how simple it can be to throw together a nourishing snack. A variety of nuts with shredded coconut provide plenty of satiating fat with a nice pop of natural sweetness from raisins and goji berries.

1. Mix all the ingredients together in a large bowl. Store in a wide-mouth mason jar for easy pouring and keep in the fridge for up to 2 months.

Farmers' Market Muffins

Makes: 10 muffins

Prep Time: 15 minutes
Cook Time: 25 to
30 minutes

Dry Ingredients

2½ cups fine almond flour

1 teaspoon baking powder

1 teaspoon ground cinnamon

¼ teaspoon ground nutmeg

¼ teaspoon ground cardamom

½ teaspoon sea salt

Wet Ingredients

1 cup loosely packed, finely grated unpeeled zucchini

¼ cup avocado oil

3 large pasture-raised eggs

½ cup loosely packed, finely grated unpeeled apple

1½ tablespoons maple syrup (optional)

½ teaspoon vanilla extract

½ cup finely chopped dates

These grain-free zucchini muffins are loaded with flavor and nutrients: They've got protein, a generous amount of fiber, and heart-healthy monounsaturated fats, making them an easy and filling snack or grab-and-go breakfast. They aren't overly sweet and won't spike your blood sugar the way store-bought muffins will.

1. Preheat the oven to 350°F. Line 10 cups of a 12-cup standard muffin tray with paper liners.

2. Combine the dry ingredients in a medium bowl.

3. Squeeze the zucchini to remove any extra liquid by pressing with a spoon in a fine strainer, or twisting in a piece of cheesecloth. Transfer the zucchini to a large bowl and add the avocado oil, eggs, apple, maple syrup (if using), and vanilla. Stir well with a fork.

4. Add the wet mixture to the dry mixture. Stir in the chopped dates until everything is well combined. Divide the batter among the 10 lined cups. Bake for 25 to 30 minutes, until the muffins are golden on top and a toothpick inserted in the middle of one comes out clean. Store in the fridge in an airtight container for up to 3 days.

Favorite Hummus

CONTRIBUTED BY GISELE BÜNDCHEN AND TOM BRADY

Makes: 4 cups

Prep Time: 10 minutes

2 (15-ounce) cans chickpeas (3 cups), plus ⅓ cup of the liquid

1 cup tahini

Juice of 3 lemons (about 5 tablespoons)

3 cloves garlic, peeled

1 teaspoon ground cumin

1 teaspoon Himalayan salt

3 tablespoons extra virgin olive oil

Generous drizzle of extra virgin olive oil and chopped fresh parsley

This classic creamy hummus was created by chef Susan Ryan Ackell for my friends Gisele Bündchen and Tom Brady; it's a favorite for fueling their active, healthy lifestyle. Try it as a dip with sliced cucumbers and seed crackers, or use it as a flavorful sauce in a lettuce wrap with sprouts, peppers, onions, and avocado.

1. Drain the chickpeas, reserving the liquid. Rinse the chickpeas, removing as much of the skins as possible (to avoid a bitter grainy hummus).

2. Place the chickpeas and the ⅓ cup chickpea liquid, the tahini, lemon juice, garlic, cumin, and salt in a food processor and blend until well combined. While blending, slowly drizzle in the olive oil and any additional liquid to create a creamy consistency.

3. Serve the hummus in a bowl with an extra drizzle of olive oil on top and parsley for garnish. Store in an airtight container in the refrigerator for up to 1 week.

Grab-and-Go Jerky

Makes: ½ pound jerky

Prep Time: 10 minutes, plus 12 hours marinating and 2 hours freezing

Cook Time: 8 to 10 hours

1 pound grass-fed beef top round, fat removed

¼ cup gluten-free tamari

1 teaspoon onion powder

1 teaspoon smoked paprika

¾ teaspoon chili powder

½ teaspoon garlic powder

½ teaspoon sea salt

I travel often, and this savory jerky is one of my favorite snacks to pack in my bag. It takes some preparation, but trust me: The taste, and the convenience of having homemade jerky around, is well worth a little planning. Grass-fed beef is an amazing source of protein, iron, and a healthy fat called conjugated linoleic acid, which encourages lean body mass, making this an excellent option when you need a quick bite between meals.

1. Place the meat in the freezer for 2 hours to firm up and make slicing easier.

2. Slice the beef as thin as possible, into about ⅛-inch-thick pieces.

3. In a small bowl, combine the tamari, onion powder, paprika, chili powder, garlic powder, and salt. Place in a shallow dish and add the meat, turning and tossing until well combined. Cover and refrigerate for 12 to 24 hours. Be sure to flip the meat at least once while marinating to evenly distribute the marinade.

4. Preheat the oven to the lowest setting, 150°F to 170°F. Line two baking sheets with parchment paper.

5. Remove the meat from the marinade, drain well, and pat dry with a paper towel. Place the meat on the lined baking sheets, arranging the slices so that none touch. Place in the oven and cook, flipping the slices every hour or so to allow for even drying, until dry to the touch. This will take up to 8 hours but may vary depending on the temperature of your oven.

6. Once fully dried, remove the jerky from the oven and allow to cool completely. Store in an airtight container at room temperature for up to 2 months.

Lemon–Poppy Seed Shortbread Bites

Makes: 20 to 22 bites

Prep Time: 10 minutes

Chill Time: 1 hour

2 cups unsweetened shredded coconut

½ cup cashew butter

¼ cup coconut oil, at room temperature

2 scoops (about 2 tablespoons) collagen powder

1 tablespoon grated lemon zest

½ teaspoon vanilla extract

Generous pinch of sea salt

1 Medjool date, chopped (optional)

1 teaspoon poppy seeds

Featuring cashew butter, vanilla, poppy seeds, and lemon, these bites are a decadent yet nourishing treat and are great to have around for a quick, healthy, grab-and-go snack. Coconut provides plenty of energy-boosting medium-chain triglycerides and collagen powder adds an extra dose of protein.

1. Combine the coconut, cashew butter, coconut oil, collagen powder, zest, vanilla, salt, and date (if using) in a food processor. Pulse several times until combined. Add the poppy seeds and pulse again until the mixture balls up, stopping to scrape the sides as needed.

2. Scoop about 1 tablespoon dough out of the food processor and use your hands to roll into a ball. Place the ball on a parchment-lined baking sheet and repeat to make about 20 balls. Cover and freeze for 1 hour, or until solid.

3. Serve frozen or lightly thawed (a few minutes at room temperature). Store extras in an airtight container in the fridge for a week, or in the freezer for several months.

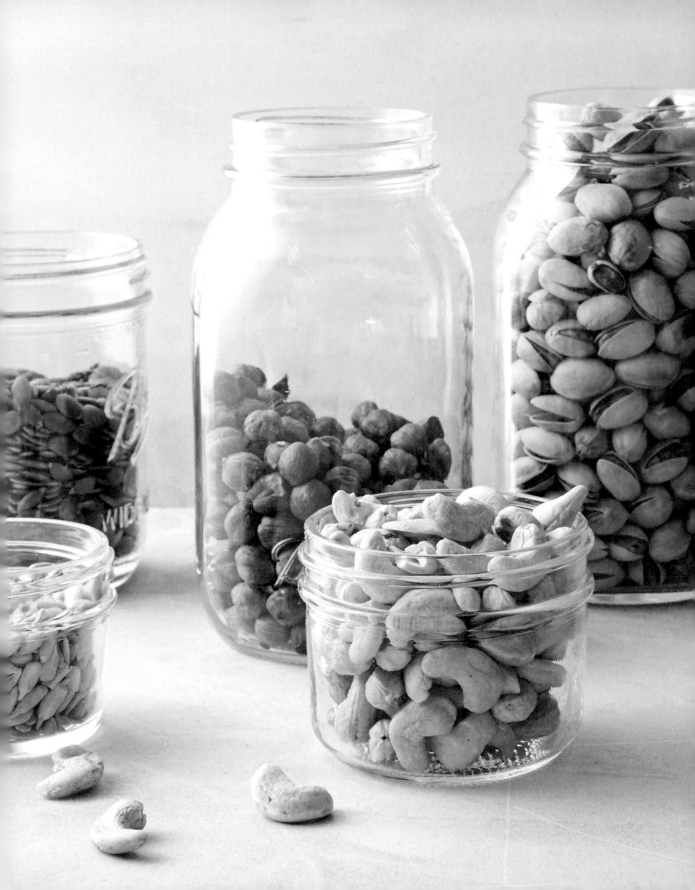

Raspberry Bliss Bars

This is an especially great snack for those of you with kids at home; they'll go crazy for the flavor combination of banana, raspberry, and coconut. And you can feel good about serving up these bars since they're full of B vitamins, minerals, fiber, and lots of healthy fats from a variety of nuts and seeds.

Makes: 16 bars

Prep Time: 15 minutes
Cook Time: 40 to
50 minutes

2 ripe bananas

⅓ cup almond butter

¼ cup nut milk
(such as almond, cashew,
or macadamia)

1 teaspoon vanilla extract

1½ cups unsweetened
shredded coconut

½ cup ground flaxseed

⅓ cup raw pepitas, chopped

⅓ cup raw sunflower seeds,
chopped

Pinch of sea salt

½ cup fresh or frozen
raspberries

1. Preheat the oven to 350°F. Line an 8 x 8-inch baking pan with parchment paper.

2. Mash the bananas in a large bowl with a fork. Stir in the almond butter, nut milk, and vanilla. Add the coconut, flaxseed, pepitas, sunflower seeds, and salt. Mix well. Break the raspberries into smaller pieces and gently fold into the banana mixture so as not to mash them.

3. Spread the batter evenly in the prepared pan. Bake for 40 to 50 minutes, until the edges are golden brown and the center is firm to the touch. Cool before slicing into 16 bars. Store extras in the fridge for up to 5 days, or wrap well and store in the freezer for a couple months.

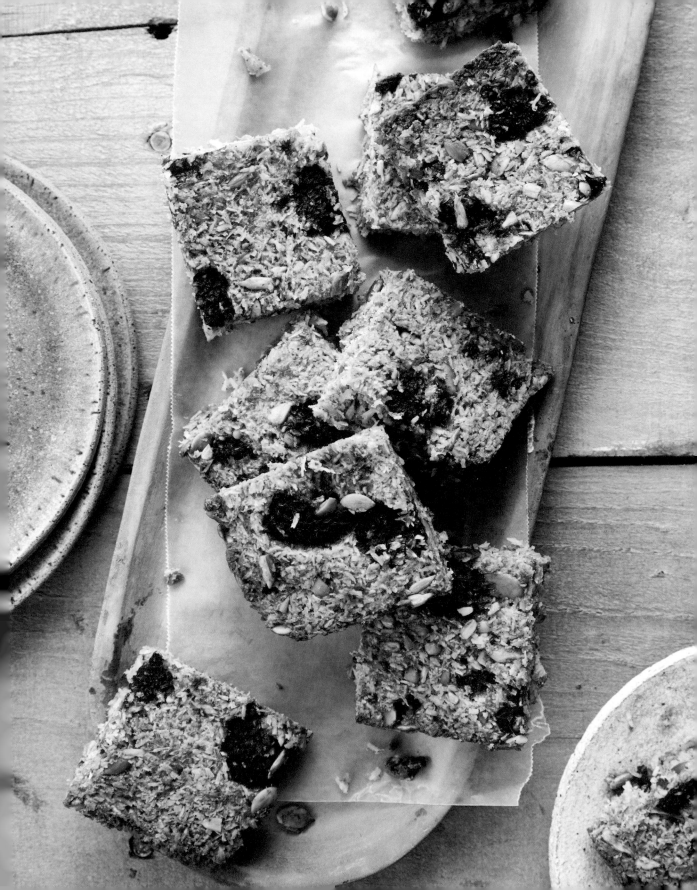

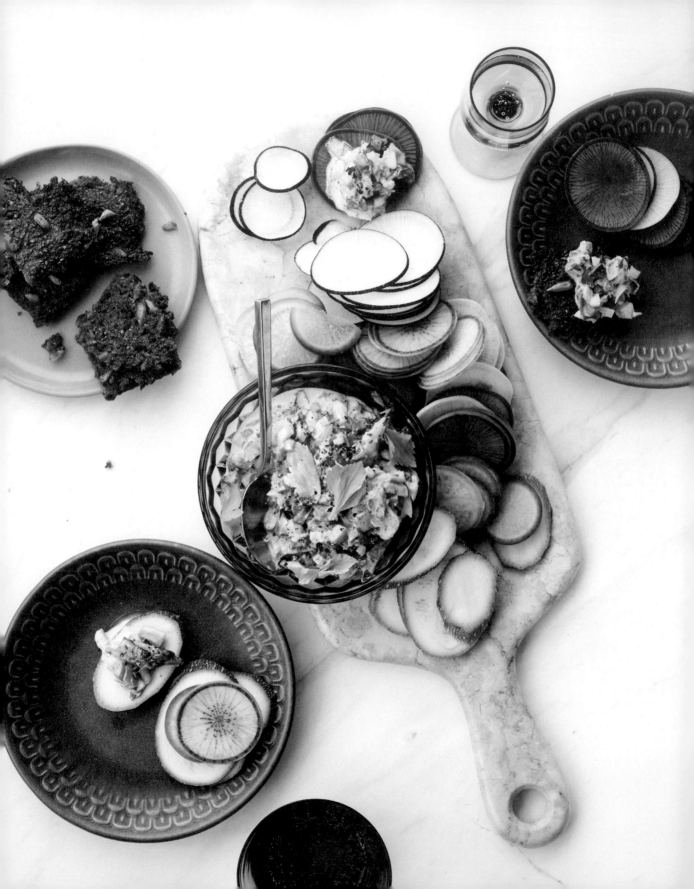

Smoked Fish Spread

Makes: 2 cups

Prep Time: 10 minutes

2 (4.4-ounce) cans lightly smoked wild-caught sardines (preferably in olive oil), drained

1 small onion, finely diced

1 small carrot, finely diced

2 celery stalks, finely diced

½ cup loosely packed fresh parsley leaves, roughly chopped

2 teaspoons onion powder

½ teaspoon garlic powder

1 teaspoon sea salt

½ cup Avocado Mayo (page 250 or store-bought)

2 tablespoons apple cider vinegar

This delicious spread is a quick and savory high-protein snack. Sardines are incredibly rich in omega-3 fatty acids and B12, making them a great choice to boost brain function. Use as a dip for veggies, spread on my Savory Seed Crackers (page 273), or spoon on top of a colorful salad.

1. In a bowl, use a fork to break the sardines into smaller pieces. Add the onion, carrot, celery, parsley, onion powder, garlic powder, and salt and stir to combine. Fold in the mayonnaise and vinegar and mix well. Store in a glass container in the fridge for up to 3 days.

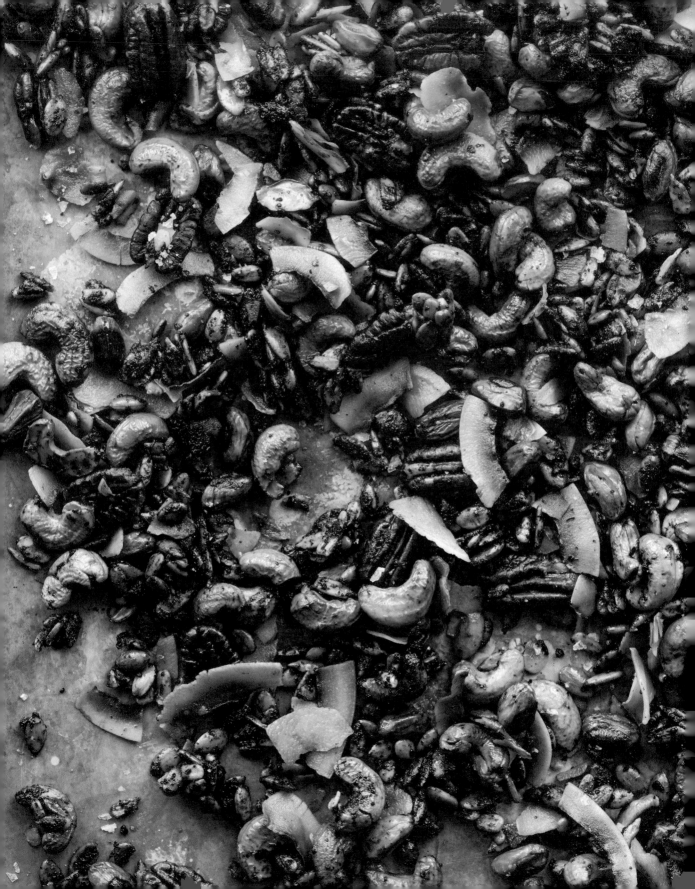

Smoky Coconut Trail Mix

It's always a good idea to keep easy, healthy options on hand so you don't reach for processed junk foods when hunger strikes. This trail mix is perfect for that and brimming with nutrients. Smoked paprika puts a unique flavor spin on the mix; it's sure to become a new favorite snack to support your active lifestyle.

Makes: 2 cups

Prep Time: 5 minutes
Cook Time: 10 minutes

½ cup raw cashews

¼ cup raw pecans

¼ cup raw pistachios

¼ cup raw pepitas

¼ cup raw sunflower seeds

2 tablespoons coconut oil or ghee

1½ teaspoons smoked paprika

¼ teaspoon garlic powder

¼ teaspoon onion powder

½ teaspoon sea salt

2 teaspoons raw honey

½ cup unsweetened flaked coconut

1. Preheat the oven to 350°F.

2. In a bowl, mix the cashews, pecans, pistachios, pepitas, and sunflower seeds. In a large pan over medium-low heat, melt the coconut oil or ghee. Add the smoked paprika, garlic powder, onion powder, and salt. Once the mixture is warm, add the honey. Turn off the heat and add the nut mixture. Mix well.

3. Spread the mixture in a single layer on a large baking sheet and bake for 7 minutes. Stir in the coconut flakes and bake for 3 minutes longer, until they are lightly toasted.

4. Let the trail mix cool completely and store in an airtight container at room temperature for up to 1 month.

Sunshine Seed Butter

Makes: 1½ cups

Prep Time: 15 minutes

2 cups raw sunflower seeds

½ cup hemp seeds

¼ cup plus 1 tablespoon coconut oil

1 tablespoon vanilla extract

1 tablespoon chia seeds

3½ teaspoons ground cinnamon

¼ teaspoon ground nutmeg

¼ teaspoon ground cardamom

¼ teaspoon sea salt

This quick and easy sunflower-based spread is sure to become a new favorite. Warming spices and nutty sunflower seeds make for a delectable, creamy spread that pairs perfectly with apples, celery, or seed crackers. It's also good right off the spoon! You're going to want to keep a jar of this in the fridge at all times.

1. Preheat the oven to 350°F. Divide the sunflower seeds among 2 baking sheets and toast in the oven for 5 minutes, until fragrant and lightly browned.

2. Place the toasted seeds and all the remaining ingredients in a high-speed blender or food processor and purée until a smooth, creamy butter is formed. Stop and scrape down the sides as necessary. This can take up to 10 minutes.

3. Scoop the butter into a jar for storage. It will last in the fridge for up to 1 month.

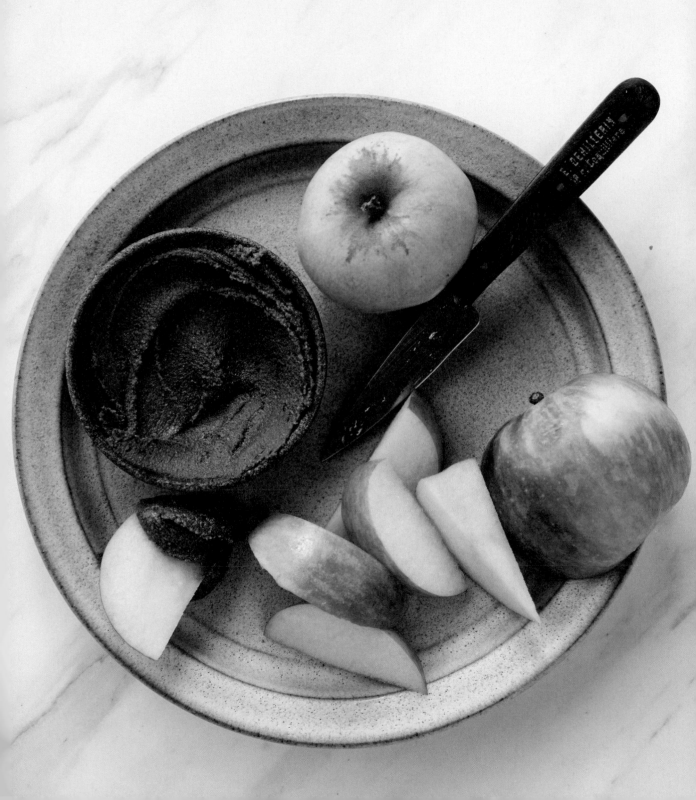

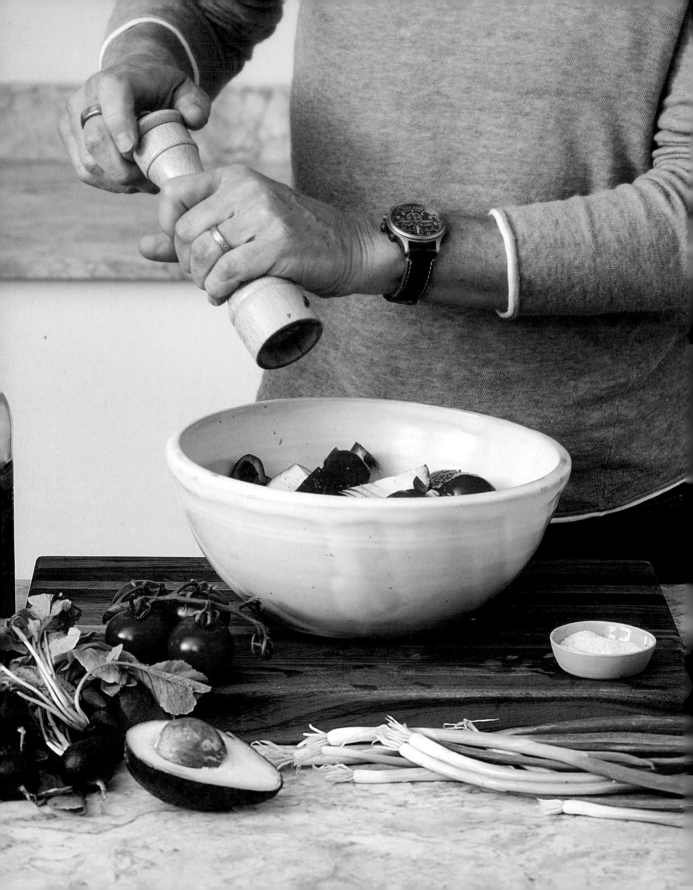

Salads

Salads are a must-have component of any healthy diet, but that doesn't mean eating the same boring one over and over again! There are so many different kinds of delicious, nutritious greens; I always keep a few different varieties on hand. Tossing them with an assortment of colorful veggies, crunchy nuts or seeds, flavorful extras like olives or fruit, and some savory protein creates a satisfying, one-bowl meal. These hearty and diverse options will keep your intake of greens high and your body happy.

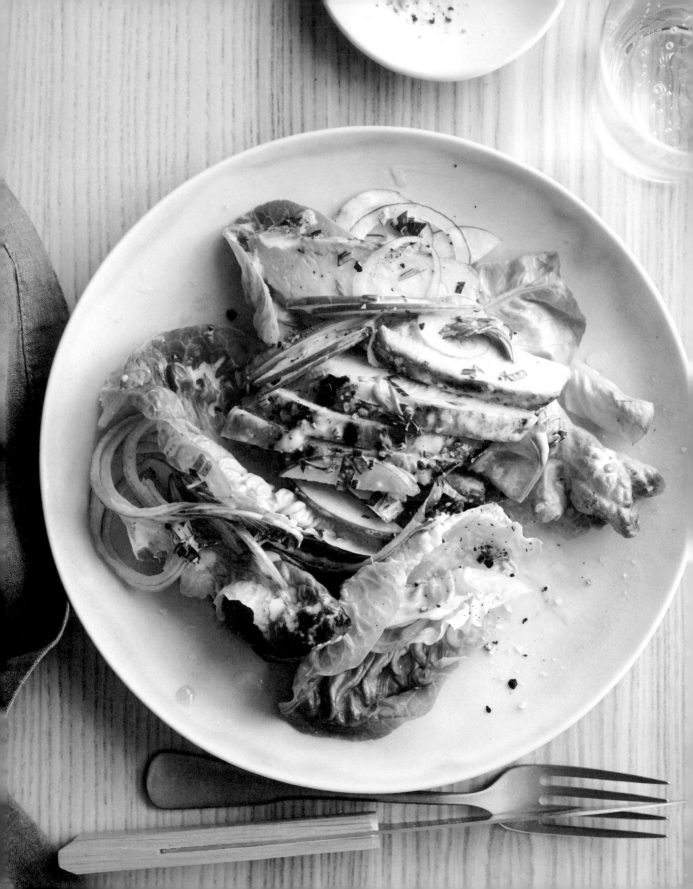

Chicken and Apple Salad

Serves: 4

Prep Time: 10 minutes
Cook Time: 10 minutes

4 large pasture-raised boneless, skinless chicken breasts

3 teaspoons sea salt

½ teaspoon freshly ground black pepper

¼ cup avocado oil

½ cup Avocado Mayo (page 250 or store-bought)

¼ cup plus 2 tablespoons lemon juice

½ cup loosely packed fresh parsley leaves, roughly chopped

2 teaspoons chopped fresh rosemary

2 large Fuji apples, cored and thinly sliced

1 small red onion, thinly sliced

6 cups mixed salad greens

¼ cup extra virgin olive oil

Crispy, juicy, and tangy, this salad is delicious for lunch or dinner—and it takes no time at all to prepare. Apples are rich in bioflavonoids, fiber, and vitamin C, and they add a natural sweetness that pairs nicely with tart lemon juice and fresh parsley.

1. Season both sides of the chicken breasts with 1 teaspoon of the salt and the pepper. In a large skillet, warm the avocado oil over medium-high heat. Add the chicken and cook for 5 minutes. Flip and continue to cook for another 4 to 5 minutes, until the meat is opaque throughout and the internal temperature reaches 165°F on an instant-read thermometer. Transfer the breasts to a cutting board and let rest for 2 minutes.

2. Cut the chicken into thin slices. In a medium bowl, combine the chicken, mayo, ¼ cup of the lemon juice, the parsley, rosemary, apple, onion, and remaining 2 teaspoons sea salt. Stir well to combine.

3. Toss the greens in a bowl with the remaining 2 tablespoons lemon juice and the olive oil, then arrange on four plates. Divide the chicken mixture evenly among the plates and serve.

Feel-Good Pesto Steak Salad

Serves: 4

Prep Time: 15 minutes
Cook Time: 20 minutes

Pesto Vinaigrette

1 cup fresh basil leaves

½ cup fresh mint leaves

3 cloves garlic, peeled

¼ cup raw pine nuts

3 tablespoons red wine vinegar

1 tablespoon Dijon mustard

½ teaspoon pink Himalayan salt or sea salt

¼ teaspoon crushed black pepper

½ cup extra virgin olive oil

Grilled Veggies

1 red bell pepper, stemmed, halved, and seeded

1 yellow bell pepper, stemmed, halved, and seeded

1 large zucchini, quartered lengthwise

1 bunch green onions, trimmed

10 radishes, halved

1 large avocado, pitted, peeled, and quartered

1 small red onion, quartered

2 fennel bulbs, cored and quartered

2 cups mixed mushrooms (such as maitake, King Trumpet, or others)

¼ cup avocado oil

½ teaspoon pink Himalayan salt or sea salt

Here's a simple, fresh, and satisfying salad full of healthy fats to boost brain health, cellular integrity, and metabolism—and it's a personal favorite that I make every week. A bright vinaigrette of basil and mint is the perfect complement to savory steak and spicy arugula. Don't forget to always choose grass-fed beef to get the most nutrition out of your animal protein. The steak and veggies can be grilled on a grill or a grill pan.

1. For the vinaigrette: Combine the basil, mint, garlic, and pine nuts in a food processor and pulse several times until a coarse mixture forms. Add the vinegar, mustard, salt, and pepper. Turn on the food processor, then slowly drizzle in the olive oil and blend until incorporated.

2. To grill the veggies: Preheat a grill or grill pan to medium-high. While the grill or grill pan is warming, prep the veggies: In a large bowl, toss the peppers, zucchini, green onions, radishes, avocado, red onion, fennel, and mushrooms with the avocado oil and salt. Place the vegetables on the grill rack or pan and grill 4 minutes on each side, or until slightly blackened. Remove the vegetables from the grill and cool slightly. Cut into 1-inch pieces and set aside.

3. To grill the steak: Heat the grill or grill pan to high. Coat the steak with the avocado oil, salt, and pepper. Grill the steak 4 minutes per side for medium-rare, or longer to desired doneness. Transfer to a cutting board and allow to rest for 2 to 3 minutes, then cut into slices.

4. To assemble the salad: In a large bowl, combine the grilled vegetables with the arugula, tomatoes, and hemp seeds. Add the vinaigrette and toss gently. Transfer the salad to a serving platter and place the steak slices on top. Garnish with a sprinkle of hemp seeds and enjoy.

Steak

1½ pound grass-fed sirloin steak

2 tablespoons avocado oil

½ teaspoon pink Himalayan salt

½ teaspoon freshly ground black pepper

Salad

2 bunches arugula

1 cup cherry tomatoes, halved

½ cup hemp seeds, plus more for garnish

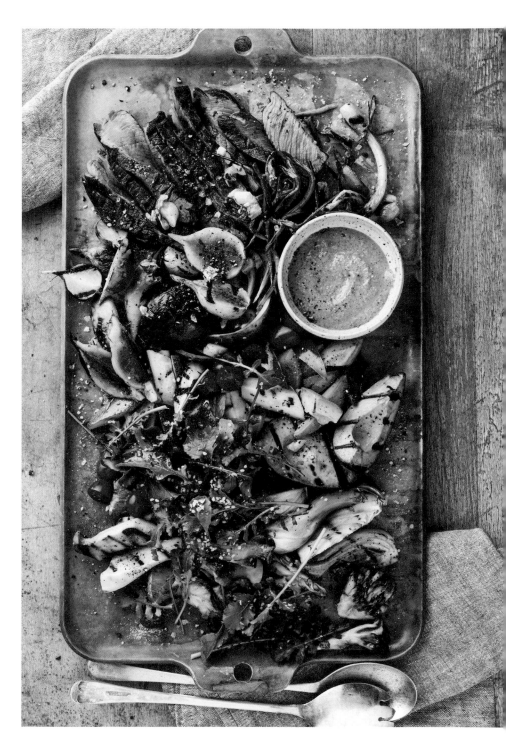

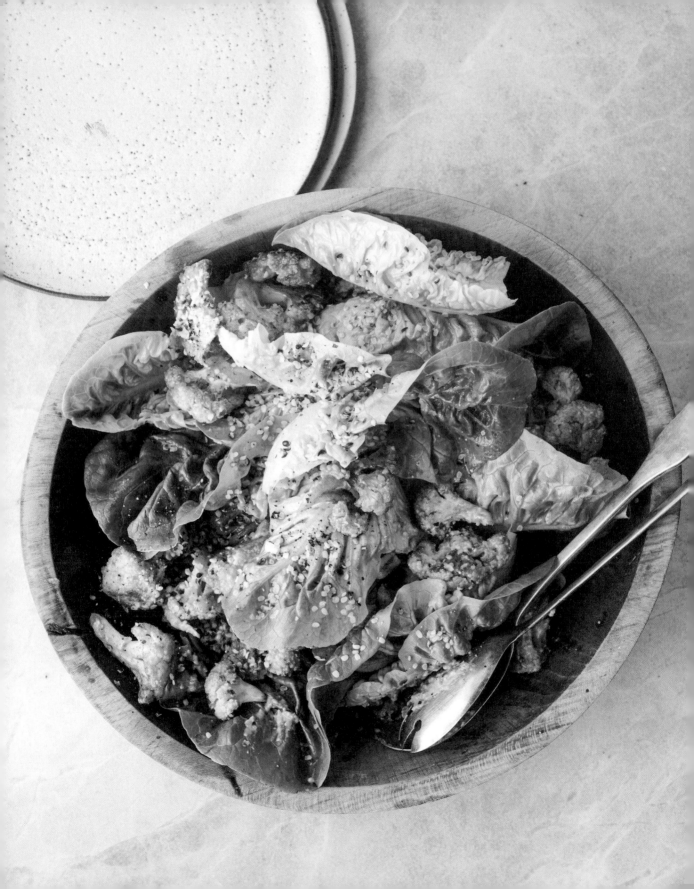

Golden Cauliflower Caesar Salad

Serves: 4

Prep Time: 15 minutes
Cook Time: 20 minutes

Roasted Cauliflower

5 cups cauliflower florets

1½ tablespoons avocado oil

1 teaspoon ground turmeric

½ teaspoon onion powder

½ teaspoon sea salt, plus more to taste

Dressing

¼ cup extra virgin olive oil

2 tablespoons Dijon mustard

1 tablespoon plus 1 teaspoon gluten-free tamari

¼ teaspoon grated lemon zest

1 tablespoon lemon juice

½ cup raw pine nuts

½ shallot, minced

2 tablespoons capers, drained and chopped

2 teaspoons pressed garlic

¼ teaspoon ground turmeric

¼ teaspoon freshly ground black pepper, plus more for seasoning

Salad

4 heads little gem lettuce, washed and leaves separated

2 tablespoons hemp seeds

4 lemon wedges

This savory salad is an amazing dairy-free alternative to a traditional Caesar. Cauliflower adds extra fiber, vitamin C, and vitamin K, and helps soak up the delicious, creamy dressing. The pine nuts in the dressing provide an extra layer of flavor and texture along with a healthy type of fat called pinolenic acid, which has been shown to support satiety hormones. The beautiful golden hue of turmeric makes this an impressive dish to serve guests that also provides anti-inflammatory benefits.

1. Preheat the oven to 375°F; line a baking sheet with parchment paper.

2. In a large mixing bowl, toss the cauliflower with the avocado oil, turmeric, onion powder, and salt. Spread the cauliflower on the lined baking sheet. Roast for 20 minutes, or until the cauliflower has started to brown and is easily pierced with a fork. Let cool slightly.

3. Meanwhile, for the dressing: Combine all ingredients in a small food processor and blend until smooth.

4. To assemble the salads: Toss the cauliflower with the dressing in a bowl. Divide the gem leaves among four plates and spoon cauliflower mixture over each bed of lettuce. Top each serving with 1½ teaspoons hemp seeds, a lemon wedge, and more sea salt and fresh pepper to taste.

Herb and Beet Boston Salad

Serves: 4

Prep Time: 20 minutes
Cook Time: 30 minutes

This salad is a beautiful blend of crisp textures and fresh flavors. Boston lettuce is a tender variety of leafy green that serves as the perfect backdrop for crisp cucumbers, radishes, and beets, all topped with a savory herb dressing. Roasted chickpeas are a healthy substitute for croutons and add extra-satisfying crunch.

1. Preheat the oven to 375°F; line a baking sheet with parchment paper.

2. To roast the chickpeas: In a large bowl, combine the chickpeas, avocado oil, onion powder, turmeric, paprika, salt, and pepper. Toss well to combine and spread out on the lined baking sheet. Roast for 15 minutes, then toss the chickpeas. Roast for an additional 15 minutes, until crispy.

3. Meanwhile make the dressing: In a medium bowl, combine the basil, mint, shallot, vinegar, sesame oil, mustard, garlic, salt, and pepper. Stir to combine, then drizzle in the olive oil. Stir well and set aside for at least 15 minutes.

4. To assemble the salad: Divide the lettuce among four bowls. Top the bowls with equal amounts of beets, cucumber, radish, avocado, pistachios, and sesame seeds. Divide the crispy chickpeas among the salads and drizzle each with dressing before serving.

Roasted Chickpeas

1 (15-ounce) can chickpeas, rinsed and drained well

1 tablespoon avocado oil

1 teaspoon onion powder

1 teaspoon ground turmeric

½ teaspoon paprika

1 teaspoon sea salt

½ teaspoon freshly ground black pepper

Herb Dressing

¼ cup fresh basil leaves, finely chopped

¼ cup fresh mint leaves, finely chopped

2 tablespoons minced shallot

2 tablespoons red wine vinegar

1 tablespoon toasted sesame oil

2 teaspoons Dijon mustard

½ teaspoon pressed garlic

¼ teaspoon sea salt

¼ teaspoon freshly ground black pepper

¼ cup extra virgin olive oil

Salad

10 cups Boston lettuce, torn into bite-size pieces

2 very small yellow beets, peeled, halved, and thinly sliced into half-moons

1 cup thinly sliced halved English cucumber

4 medium radishes, thinly sliced into half-moons

1 avocado, pitted, peeled, and thinly sliced

¼ cup raw pistachios, finely chopped

2 tablespoons white sesame seeds

Kale, Carrot, and Avo Salad with Tahini Dressing

CONTRIBUTED BY GWYNETH PALTROW

Serves: 4

Prep Time: 10 minutes

4 small shallots, minced

4 cloves garlic, grated

½ cup tahini

½ cup filtered water

Juice of 1 lemon

2 tablespoons apple cider vinegar

½ teaspoon kosher salt

4 cups thinly sliced black kale

2 cups grated carrots

2 avocados, pitted, peeled, and thinly sliced

½ cup toasted sunflower seeds

This refreshing, nutrient-dense salad comes from my friend Gwyneth Paltrow's latest book, *The Clean Plate: Eat, Reset, Heal.* Black kale, also known as Tuscan or lacinato kale, is an incredible source of isothiocyanates, plant compounds with anticancer, neuro-protective, and immune-modulating properties. It creates a crisp base for a rich and creamy tahini dressing that I know you'll love as much as I do.

1. Mix the shallots, garlic, tahini, water, lemon juice, vinegar, and salt in a jar until well combined.

2. Toss the kale and carrots in a large serving bowl. Drizzle with the dressing, then top with avocado and sunflower seeds to serve.

Roasted Veggies and Pepitas

1 medium sweet potato, peeled and cut into small wedges about ¼-inch thick

2 cups chopped purple cabbage

2 tablespoons avocado oil

½ teaspoon ground cumin

¼ teaspoon chili powder

¼ teaspoon garlic powder

¼ teaspoon smoked paprika

½ teaspoon sea salt

¼ cup pepitas

Salsa

2 medium tomatoes, seeded and finely diced (about 1⅓ cups)

½ small white onion, finely diced (½ cup)

½ cup tightly packed fresh cilantro, finely chopped

¼ cup lime juice

¼ cup extra virgin olive oil

1½ teaspoons pressed garlic

¼ teaspoon ground cumin

½ teaspoon sea salt

Chicken

4 small pasture-raised boneless, skinless chicken breasts (about 1¼ pounds)

1 tablespoon avocado oil

¼ teaspoon onion powder

¼ teaspoon smoked paprika

½ teaspoon sea salt, plus more for seasoning

¼ teaspoon freshly ground black pepper

Mexican Chicken Salad

Roasted sweet potatoes and cabbage combine with spinach and juicy chicken to create this filling salad. I enjoy it as a nourishing one-bowl meal for lunch or dinner. It provides plenty of phytonutrients from colorful veggies, along with protein from chicken and good fats from pumpkin seeds and avocado. You can make this ahead of time, just keep the salsa separate until you're ready to serve.

1. Preheat the oven to 350°F; line a baking sheet with parchment paper.

2. For the roasted veggies: Combine the sweet potatoes, cabbage, avocado oil, cumin, chili powder, garlic powder, paprika, and salt in a large bowl. Arrange on the lined baking sheet, making sure the veggies are spread out evenly. Roast for 35 minutes, or until the sweet potatoes are fork-tender. Transfer to a bowl.

3. For the pepitas: Spread on a separate, unlined baking sheet. Bake in the oven for 5 minutes, until toasted. Remove from oven and set aside.

4. For the salsa: In a bowl, combine the tomatoes, onion, cilantro, lime juice, olive oil, garlic, cumin, and salt. Allow the salsa to sit for at least 15 minutes before serving.

5. For the chicken: Rub the chicken breasts with the avocado oil, onion powder, paprika, salt, and pepper. Place on the parchment-lined baking sheet used for the sweet potatoes and cabbage and transfer to the oven. Roast for 15 minutes, then flip the chicken and roast for another 15 minutes or so, until the internal temperature of the meat is 165°F. Let the chicken cool slightly, then tear into bite-size pieces.

6. To assemble the salad: In a large salad bowl, combine the roasted veggies, toasted pepitas, salsa, chicken, and spinach. Divide among four bowls and top with the avocado, a lime wedge, and sea salt to taste.

Salad

10 ounces baby spinach, roughly chopped

1 avocado, pitted, peeled, and chopped

1 lime, quartered

Sticky Pomegranate Chicken Salad

CONTRIBUTED BY RUPY AUJLA, MD

Serves: 4

Prep Time: 5 minutes
Cook Time: 20 minutes

½ cup extra virgin olive oil, plus more for drizzling

2 tablespoons tomato paste

2 tablespoons pomegranate molasses (or maple syrup or honey), optional

4 large cloves garlic, minced

¼ cup ground sumac

2 teaspoons dried oregano

1 teaspoon red chili flakes

4 pasture-raised boneless, skinless chicken thighs

1 medium red onion, thinly sliced

⅔ cup raw hazelnuts, chopped

8 cups arugula

4 cups cooked Puy or green lentils

This unique, flavorful recipe comes from my good friend Dr. Rupy Aujla, the author of one of my favorite cookbooks, *The Doctor's Kitchen*. Sumac is a spice with a bright, lemony flavor that is used in traditional Middle Eastern cooking. It's the perfect complement to sweet pomegranate molasses and spicy arugula. This salad has all your nutritional needs covered with plenty of protein from chicken, fiber from lentils, beneficial monounsaturated fats from olive oil, and lots of phytonutrients from the spices, hazelnuts, and greens.

1. Preheat the oven to 400°F.

2. Combine the olive oil, tomato paste, pomegranate molasses, garlic, sumac, oregano, and chili flakes in a large bowl. Add the chicken and turn to coat with the marinade. Add the onions and mix in.

3. Transfer the chicken and onions to a baking sheet. Bake for 20 minutes, until the chicken is cooked through and browned; a meat thermometer should read 165°F.

4. Meanwhile, toast the hazelnuts in a dry pan over medium heat for 2 to 3 minutes, until lightly browned.

5. To assemble the salad, in a serving bowl toss together the arugula, lentils, a drizzle of olive oil, and the hazelnuts. Cut the chicken into ½-inch-thick slices. Top the salad with the chicken and onions and serve.

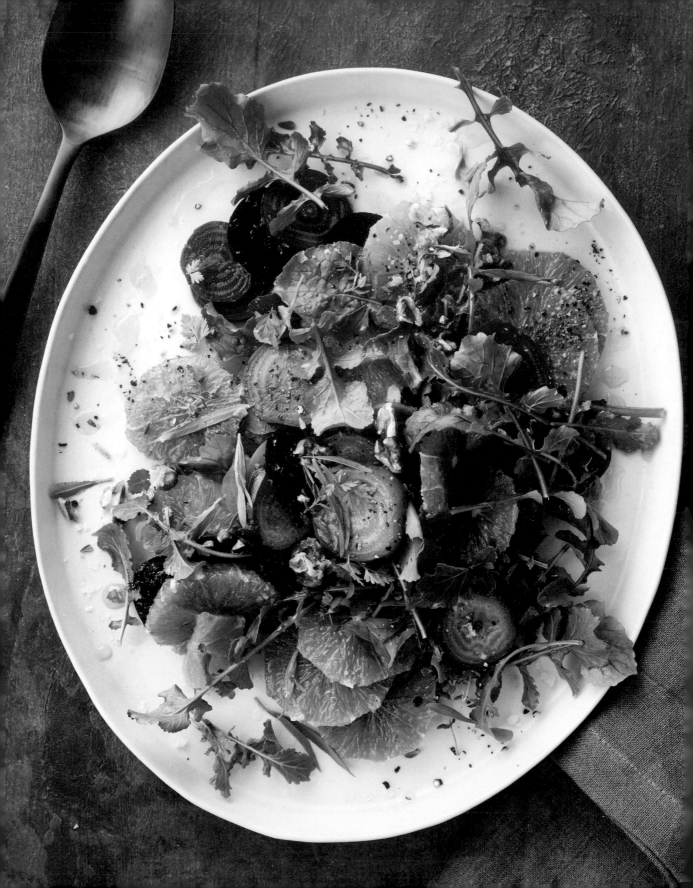

Roasted Beet and Citrus Salad

The natural sweetness of roasted beets combines with tangy citrus and spicy arugula to make this salad incredibly bright, fresh, and flavorful. Beets are full of powerful antioxidants that fight inflammation and support detoxification. The deeply colored red ones contain betalain, a unique compound that contributes to these benefits. Golden beets, on the other hand, are a great source of beta-carotene and potassium.

Serves: 4

Prep Time: 15 minutes
Cook Time: 1 hour

2 medium red beets

2 medium golden beets

½ cup raw walnuts

6 Valencia oranges
(or a mix of other types,
like navel and blood)

¼ cup plus 2 tablespoons
extra virgin olive oil

2 teaspoons chopped
fresh thyme

½ teaspoon sea salt

¼ teaspoon freshly ground
black pepper

8 cups baby arugula

1. Preheat the oven to 350°F.

2. Place the beets in a glass baking dish or Dutch oven. Add 1 cup water and cover. Roast for 1 hour, until the beets can be easily pierced with a knife or toothpick. Let cool completely.

3. Meanwhile, spread the walnuts on an ungreased baking sheet and toast in the oven for 5 minutes, or until fragrant. Let cool, then roughly chop and set aside.

4. Use your hands to remove the skins from the beets, then cut off the tops and bottoms. Slice the beets into thin rounds, about ⅛-inch thick, and set aside.

5. Peel 4 of the oranges and cut into rounds: Cut off the tops and bottoms. Stand one orange on a cut end and, using a sharp knife, pare away the rind and white pith in strips from top to bottom, following the contour of the fruit. Lay the orange on its side and cut into ¼-inch-thick rounds, yielding 6 to 8 slices. Repeat with the remaining trimmed oranges.

6. Grate the zest from the remaining 2 oranges into a small bowl. Cut the oranges in half and squeeze the juice into the same bowl. Whisk in the olive oil, thyme, salt, and pepper to make the dressing.

7. Place the arugula in a bowl and toss with ¼ cup of the dressing. Arrange the dressed greens on a platter, then lay the beets and oranges on top in an alternating pattern. Sprinkle with the toasted walnuts and drizzle with additional dressing.

Superfood Slaw

Serves: 4

Prep Time: 15 minutes, plus 30 minutes soaking

Cook Time: 5 minutes

1 cup dried wakame seaweed flakes

¼ cup raw sunflower seeds

1½ tablespoons gluten-free tamari

4½ tablespoons toasted sesame oil

2 tablespoons lime juice

3 medium green apples, unpeeled, cored, and finely diced (about 2 cups)

4 cups chopped purple cabbage

¼ cup hemp seeds

¼ cup extra virgin olive oil

2 tablespoons filtered water

2 tablespoons rice wine vinegar

1 teaspoon ume plum vinegar

1 tablespoon plus 1 teaspoon micro-grated peeled fresh ginger

1 teaspoon onion powder

½ teaspoon garlic powder

½ teaspoon sea salt

½ teaspoon freshly ground black pepper

1 avocado, pitted, peeled, quartered lengthwise, and sliced

This unique cabbage slaw is an ultra-flavorful way to get more sea vegetables into your diet. Wakame is a brown or deep green seaweed that is rich in calcium and magnesium as well as compounds that fight diabetes and obesity. Combining slightly salty wakame with tangy green apple and crunchy cabbage creates a tasty variety of colors, flavors, and textures.

1. Soak the seaweed in water for 30 minutes, then strain and squeeze well.

2. Heat a medium sauté pan over medium-high heat. Add the sunflower seeds and toast, continuously stirring and shaking, until fragrant and toasted, about 5 minutes. Remove from the heat and set aside.

3. In a medium bowl, mix the seaweed with the tamari and 2½ table-spoons of the sesame oil.

4. In a separate large bowl, pour the lime juice over the diced apples to keep them from browning. Mix in the purple cabbage and seaweed.

5. In a small food processor or blender, combine the remaining 2 table-spoons sesame oil, the hemp seeds, olive oil, water, rice wine vinegar, ume vinegar, ginger, onion powder, garlic powder, salt, and pepper. Blend until smooth.

6. Stir the dressing into the apple mixture, top with the toasted sunflower seeds and avocado, and serve.

Tahini Rainbow Cabbage Salad

Serves: 4

Prep Time: 20 minutes
Cook Time: 15 minutes

Eggs

8 large pasture-raised eggs

1 tablespoon extra virgin olive oil

½ teaspoon sea salt

¼ teaspoon freshly ground black pepper

Tahini Dressing

¼ cup tahini

3 tablespoons extra virgin olive oil

2 tablespoons filtered water

1 tablespoon plus 1 teaspoon lemon juice

1 tablespoon plus 1 teaspoon gluten-free tamari or coconut aminos

2 teaspoons pressed garlic

¼ teaspoon freshly ground black pepper

Salad

2 cups shredded purple cabbage

3 cups finely chopped spinach

1 cup finely diced red bell pepper

1 cup grated carrots

¼ cup plus 2 tablespoons finely chopped fresh cilantro

1 avocado, pitted, peeled, and chopped

¾ cup crumbled goat feta cheese

I love the crunch and natural sweetness of purple cabbage. Its beautiful color is a sign of powerful antioxidants called anthocyanins, which are especially beneficial for the cardiovascular and neurological systems. A variety of colorful vegetables, a creamy tahini dressing, and hard-boiled eggs create a salad that is a complete meal, sure to leave you feeling satisfied.

1. For the eggs: Prepare a medium bowl of ice water. Bring a medium pot of water to a boil over high heat. Gently add the eggs and boil for 13 minutes. Immediately plunge the eggs into the ice bath and let sit for 5 minutes. Gently tap the eggs on the counter to crack, then peel each and cut in half. In a bowl, gently mix the egg halves with the olive oil, salt, and pepper.

2. For the dressing: Combine all the ingredients in a jar and mix until fully blended.

3. To assemble the salad: Combine the cabbage, spinach, bell pepper, carrots, and cilantro in a large salad bowl and toss to combine. Just before serving, add the dressing and massage the salad until well combined. Add the eggs, avocado, and feta, gently turning the mixture once to lightly coat with dressing.

Toasted-Caper and Salmon Salad

Smoked wild-caught salmon is a delicious and easy way to get high-quality protein and omega-3s into your diet. In this recipe I toss it with fresh parsley and top it with a dollop of creamy cashew sauce. Toasted capers create a salty, crunchy contrast to the smoky flavor of the fish, and I love the bright finish from a squeeze of lemon juice.

Serves: 4

Prep Time: 20 minutes, plus 4 hours soaking

Cook Time: 1 minute

2 small watermelon radishes

2 tablespoons apple cider vinegar

½ cup plus 2 tablespoons avocado oil

½ teaspoon sea salt

½ teaspoon freshly ground black pepper

½ cup raw cashews, soaked 4 hours or overnight

½ cup filtered water

¼ cup nonpareil capers, rinsed and drained well

2 cups fresh parsley leaves

6 ounces smoked wild-caught salmon, cut into 2-inch pieces

Grated zest of 2 lemons

2 lemons, sliced into 6 wedges each

1. Peel and julienne the watermelon radishes. Transfer to a large bowl, add the vinegar and 2 tablespoons of the avocado oil, and toss. Mix in the salt and pepper and toss well. Let stand for 15 minutes.

2. Drain and rinse the soaked cashews. Add to a blender with the water. Blend on high for 45 seconds to 1 minute, until creamy and free of lumps.

3. Heat the remaining ½ cup avocado oil in a small pan over medium-high heat. When the oil is shimmering, carefully add the capers and cook until golden brown, 30 to 45 seconds. With a slotted spoon, transfer the capers to a plate lined with a paper towel to drain. Reserve the leftover oil and allow to cool.

4. Toss the parsley with ¼ cup of the cooled caper oil. Transfer the parsley to the bowl with the marinated radishes, add the salmon, and toss gently.

5. Arrange the salad among four plates, then top with the toasted capers and a dollop of the cashew cream. Sprinkle with the lemon zest and serve the salads with lemon wedges.

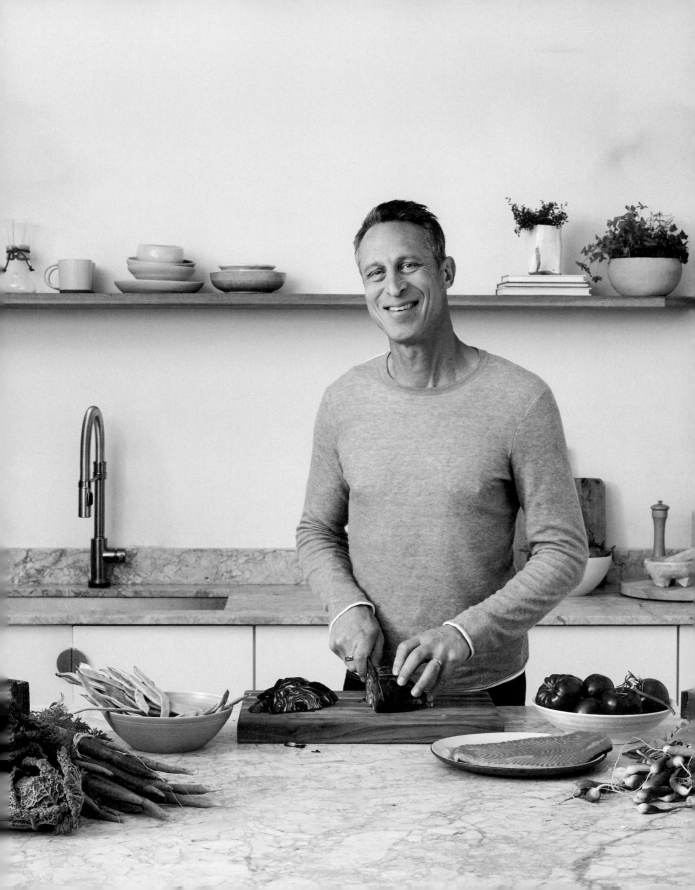

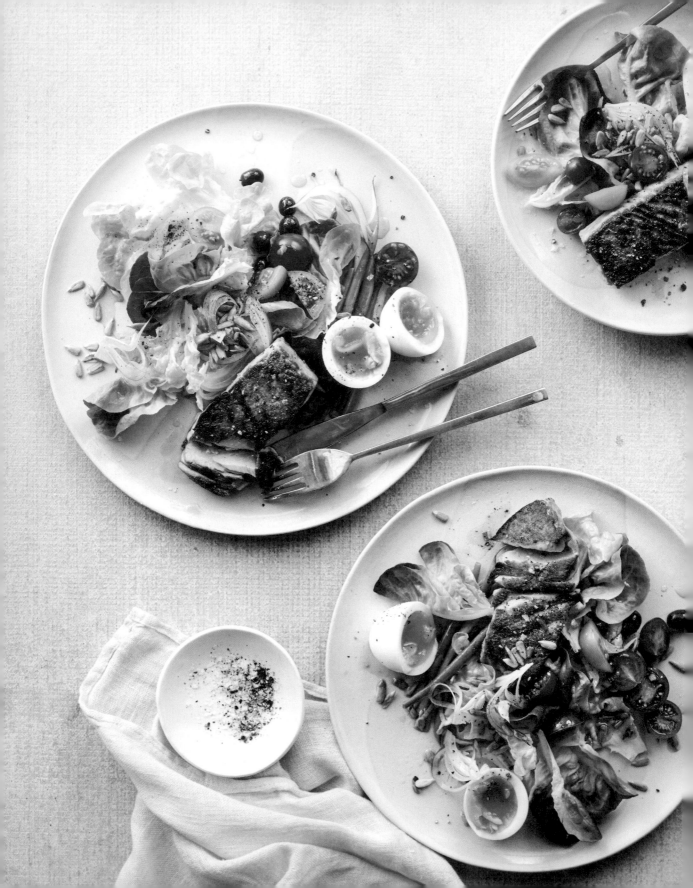

Wild Salmon Niçoise Salad

Serves: 4

Prep Time: 10 minutes

Cook Time: 20 minutes

4 large pasture-raised eggs

4 (4-ounce) wild-caught salmon fillets

1 teaspoon sea salt

¼ cup avocado oil

8 ounces salad greens

¼ cup extra virgin olive oil

2 tablespoons lemon juice

24 black olives

2 small red onions, thinly sliced

12 to 16 pickled green beans (also called dilly beans)

20 cherry tomatoes, halved

¼ cup raw sunflower seeds

This light and easy salad is a classic French favorite. Flaky salmon and hard-boiled eggs provide plenty of omega-3 fats and protein, while black olives offer antioxidant vitamin E and monounsaturated fats that benefit the cardiovascular system. This is a quick but tasty meal to whip up for lunch or a weeknight dinner.

1. Prepare a medium bowl of ice water. Bring a medium pot of water to a boil over high heat. Gently add eggs and boil for 13 minutes. Immediately plunge the eggs into the ice bath and let sit for 5 minutes. Gently tap the eggs on the counter to crack, then peel each and cut in half.

2. Season both sides of the salmon fillets with salt. Heat the avocado oil in a 10-inch skillet over medium-high heat. Once the oil is shimmering, add the fish, skin side up, and sear for 3 minutes. Flip the fillets and cook an additional 3 minutes, until opaque. Turn off the heat and let stand for 1 minute.

3. Place the salad greens in a bowl and toss with olive oil and lemon juice. Divide among four plates, then arrange the olives, onions, pickled beans, tomatoes, and sunflower seeds evenly on top of the greens. Add the eggs and salmon and serve.

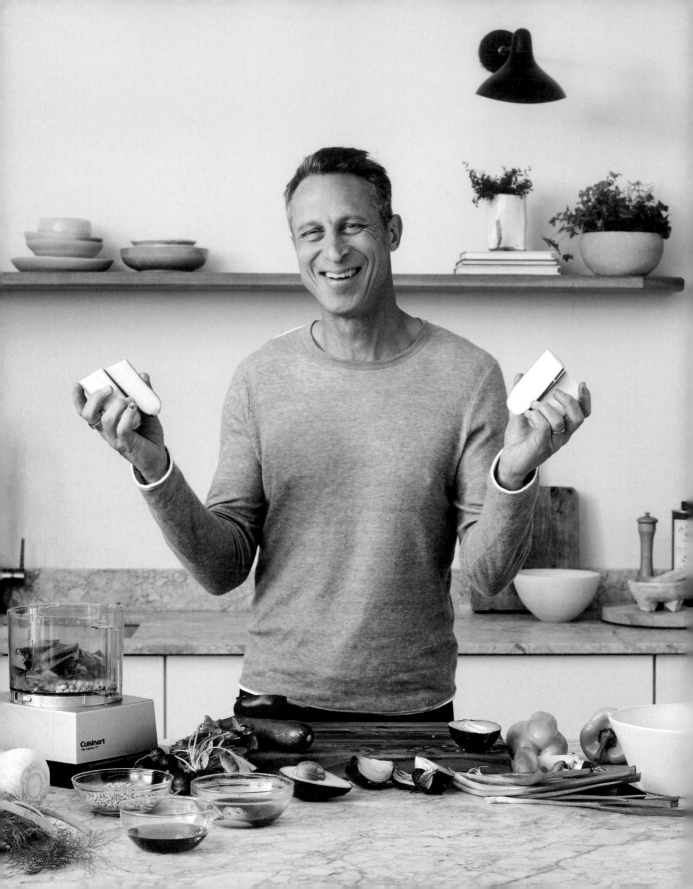

Soups and Stews

Soups and stews are a comforting, nutrient-dense addition to any diet. The possibilities of flavors, textures, colors, and aromas are endless, and I often find myself using whatever I have on hand to make one big, warm, delicious pot that can feed both my wife and me for a couple days. Try pairing the dishes in this section with some of my salads and sides for a satiating and beautiful meal.

African Sweet Potato Stew

CONTRIBUTED BY HUGH JACKMAN

This satisfying stew was shared by my friend Hugh Jackman. It's one of his favorites from the handwritten cookbook his mother made for him. I love to eat plenty of garlic, ginger, and cayenne during the colder months to boost my immune system, and this stew has all that and more. Sweet potatoes, mushrooms, and spinach add an extra dose of colorful nutrients and delicious flavors.

Serves: 4

Prep Time: 15 minutes
Cook Time: 45 minutes

¼ cup extra virgin olive oil

1 medium onion, chopped

2 cloves garlic, minced

2 teaspoons grated peeled fresh ginger

½ teaspoon cayenne pepper

1 tablespoon mild curry paste

1 medium sweet potato (about ¾ pound), peeled and chopped into ½-inch pieces

1¼ cups vegetable broth

1 (28-ounce) can diced tomatoes

2 cups button mushrooms

1 heaping cup baby spinach, chopped

3 tablespoons peanut butter

2 tablespoons chopped fresh cilantro, plus more for garnish

Sea salt and freshly ground black pepper

1. Heat the olive oil in a large pot over medium heat until shimmering. Add the onion, garlic, ginger, and cayenne and cook gently for 10 minutes. Add the curry paste, stir well, and cook for 1 minute. Stir in the sweet potato and cook for another 3 to 4 minutes. Add the broth and tomatoes and bring to a boil. Cover, reduce the heat, and simmer for 15 to 20 minutes, until the sweet potato is fork-tender. Add the mushrooms and cook for another 5 minutes, then stir in the spinach.

2. In a small bowl, mix a couple scoops of stew with the peanut butter and stir well, then mix this back into the stew. Stir in the cilantro and add salt and pepper to taste.

3. To serve, ladle the stew into bowls and garnish with additional cilantro.

Mediterranean Lentil Stew

Serves: 6

Prep Time: 20 minutes
Cook Time: 40 minutes

1 cup split red lentils

2 tablespoons avocado oil

1 large white onion, chopped (about 1½ cups)

1 medium carrot, peeled and chopped (about 1 cup)

1 tablespoon pressed garlic

Grated zest of 1 lemon

1 bunch green kale, stemmed and shredded

1 (28-ounce) can chopped tomatoes

1½ teaspoons dried oregano

1½ teaspoons dried basil

1 teaspoon dried thyme

1 teaspoon garlic powder

2 teaspoons sea salt, plus more for seasoning

4 cups (32 ounces) vegetable broth

1 medium zucchini, chopped (about 1½ cups)

2 tablespoons lemon juice

Freshly ground black pepper

4 ounces goat cheese (optional)

This hearty stew is an aromatic blend of herbs and spices cooked with red lentils and a variety of tasty vegetables. Onions, carrots, kale, and zucchini provide lots of fiber and nutrients, like prebiotics, beta-carotene, and vitamin C. Oregano is a staple in Mediterranean cooking and one of my personal favorites; it's naturally antibacterial and contains several types of antioxidants while lending a warm and slightly sweet flavor.

1. Rinse the lentils until the water runs clear; set aside to drain in a sieve.

2. Heat the avocado oil in a large pot over medium heat. When the oil is shimmering, add the onion and sauté until translucent, about 5 minutes. Add the carrot, pressed garlic, and lemon zest and stir well for 3 minutes.

3. Add the drained lentils, kale, tomatoes, oregano, basil, thyme, garlic powder, and salt and stir well for 1 minute. Add the broth and bring the mixture to a boil over high heat. Reduce the heat, cover, and simmer for 20 minutes, or until the lentils are cooked through, stirring occasionally.

4. Add the zucchini and lemon juice and cook over medium-low heat for another 10 minutes. Season with more salt if needed and black pepper to taste.

5. Serve warm with dollops of goat cheese, if desired.

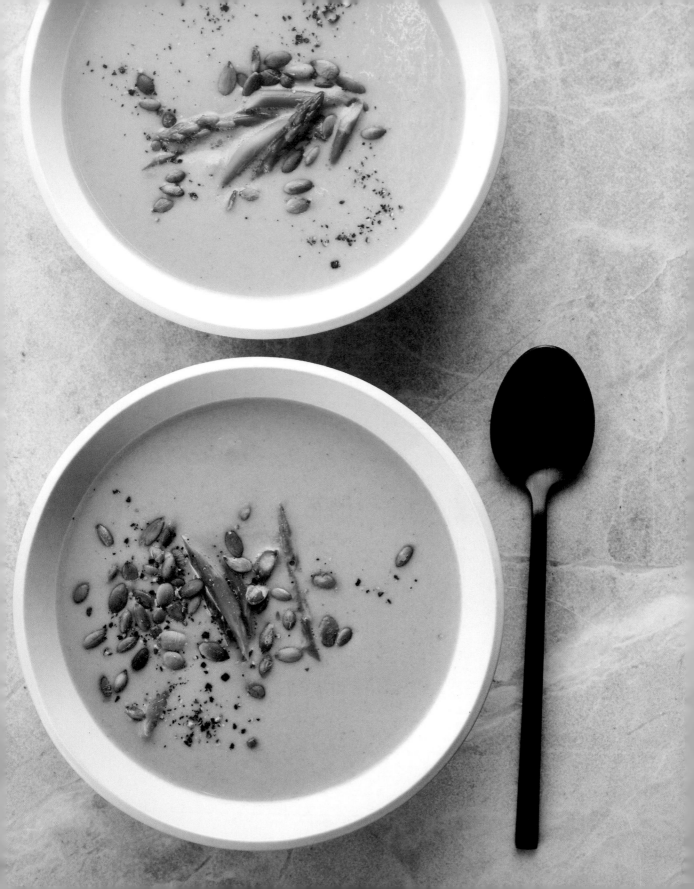

Anti-Aging Asparagus Soup

Serves: 4

Prep Time: 15 minutes
Cook Time: 20 minutes

2 bunches asparagus

¼ cup pepitas

3 tablespoons plus 1 teaspoon avocado oil

1 medium white onion, finely diced

2 tablespoons micro-grated peeled fresh ginger

3½ large leeks, chopped

3 tablespoons coconut aminos

4 cups (32 ounces) vegetable broth

1 teaspoon smoked paprika

1 teaspoon garlic powder

½ teaspoon sea salt

Grated zest of 1 lemon

1 cup full-fat unsweetened coconut milk

4 scoops (about ¼ cup) collagen powder (optional, not vegan friendly)

Freshly ground black pepper

This soup makes an excellent meal all on its own, thanks to healthy fats from coconut milk, protein from healing collagen powder, and phytonutrients from asparagus, leeks, and garlic. Those benefits also make it a great way to fight the aging process and support a resilient body. It's creamy and filling with just the right amount of spice from fresh ginger and smoked paprika, though you can use less of these ingredients if you prefer.

1. Cut 4 of the asparagus spears into thirds and set aside for garnish. Roughly chop the remaining spears.

2. Heat a medium sauté pan over medium-high heat. Add the pepitas and continuously stir and shake until the seeds are fragrant and toasted, about 5 minutes. Remove from the heat and set aside.

3. Heat the 3 tablespoons avocado oil in a large pot over medium heat until shimmering. Add the onion and sauté for 5 minutes. Add the ginger, leeks, and coconut aminos, stir well, and cook down for 5 minutes. Add the chopped asparagus, broth, paprika, garlic powder, and salt and bring the mixture to a boil over medium heat. Reduce the heat and add the lemon zest and coconut milk.

4. Remove the soup from the heat and allow to cool for several minutes. Pour into a blender, add the collagen powder (if using), and blend until smooth.

5. Heat the remaining 1 teaspoon avocado oil in a small sauté pan over medium-high until shimmering. Add the reserved asparagus spears and lightly sauté until tender, about 3 minutes.

6. To serve, divide the soup among four bowls and place 3 pieces of sautéed asparagus in the center of each bowl. Sprinkle with the toasted pepitas and freshly ground pepper.

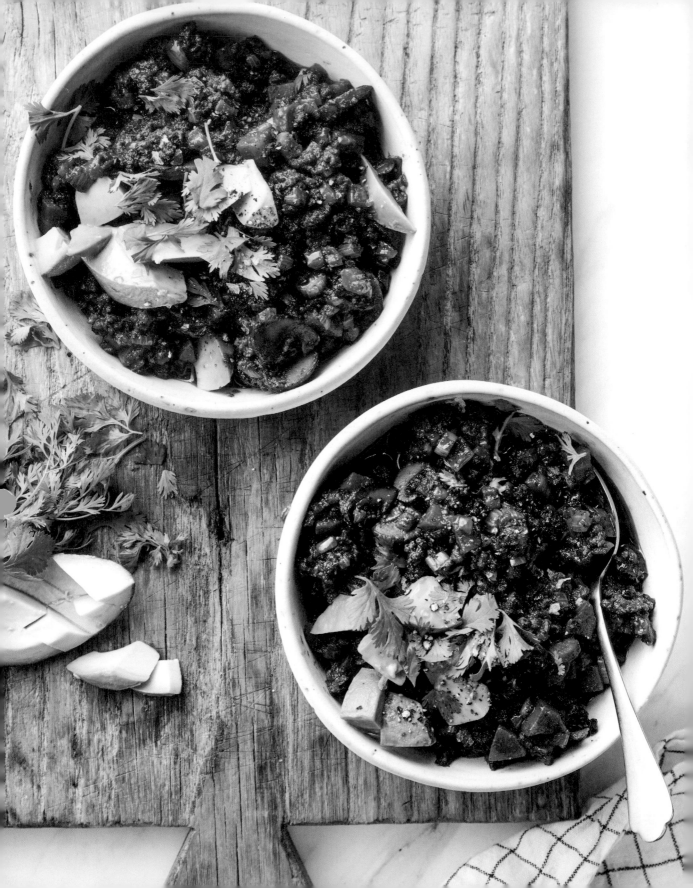

Go-To Cremini Chili

Serves: 4

Prep Time: 15 minutes
Cook Time: 55 minutes

2 tablespoons ghee or
coconut oil

1 pound grass-fed ground
beef (optional)

12 large cremini mushrooms
(24 if you forgo the beef),
roughly chopped

2 large red onions,
roughly chopped

2 large carrots,
roughly chopped

2 red bell peppers, stemmed,
seeded, and roughly chopped

4 celery stalks, roughly
chopped

4 cloves garlic, minced

2 tablespoons chili powder

1 tablespoon plus 1 teaspoon
dried oregano

2 teaspoons garlic powder

½ teaspoon chipotle powder

1 (15-ounce) can tomato purée

6 cups filtered water

¼ teaspoon sea salt

1 large avocado, pitted, peeled,
and sliced

½ cup loosely packed fresh
cilantro leaves, roughly
chopped

Everyone needs a go-to chili recipe. This one puts a tasty spin on classic flavors by adding tender cremini mushrooms, which you can double to make a meat-free version. Chili powder, oregano, garlic, and chipotle powder create a spicy and savory base while providing cardiovascular and metabolic benefits. I love eating leftover chili for lunch; store any extra in the fridge in an airtight container for up to 3 days.

1. Heat a 6-quart Dutch oven over medium-high heat, add the ghee, and heat until shimmering. If using, add the beef and cook, using a wooden spoon to break it up into small pieces and allowing the meat to sear and brown for about 3 minutes.

2. Add the mushrooms, onions, carrots, bell peppers, and celery, stirring well to combine. Cook until the vegetables are soft, 4 to 5 minutes.

3. Add the minced garlic, chili powder, oregano, garlic powder, and chipotle powder and stir well. Add the tomato purée and water and bring to a boil. Cover, reduce the heat to medium, and cook slowly until the chili has reduced and thickened, about 45 minutes.

4. Finish the chili by seasoning with the salt. Divide among four bowls and top with avocado and chopped cilantro.

Soul Food Yam Soup

Serves: 4

Prep Time: 20 minutes
Cook Time: 35 minutes

2 tablespoons avocado oil

½ cup chopped fresh cilantro

1 large sweet onion, chopped (about 2 cups)

1 tablespoon pressed garlic

1½ teaspoons ground cumin

¼ teaspoon chili powder

1 medium garnet yam, unpeeled, chopped (about 2 cups)

1 small head cauliflower, chopped (about 2 cups)

4 cups filtered water

1 teaspoon garlic powder

½ teaspoon onion powder

¼ teaspoon smoked paprika

1 large lime, peeled

¼ cup tahini

1 teaspoon sea salt

4 cups spinach, finely chopped, plus more for garnish

¼ cup thinly sliced green onions

2½ tablespoons black sesame seeds

This rich, creamy soup is the ultimate warm, comforting meal for a cold day. When blended with tahini, tangy lime, and plenty of savory spices, the cauliflower and yam take on a smooth texture to create a filling soup rich in beta-carotene, calcium, and immune-boosting phytonutrients. I love to enjoy this soup with my Feel-Good Pesto Steak Salad (page 118).

1. Heat the avocado oil in a large pot over medium until shimmering. Add the cilantro and onion, stir well, and cook down for 6 minutes. Add the garlic, cumin, and chili powder and stir well for 1 minute.

2. Add the yam, cauliflower, water, garlic powder, onion powder, and paprika and bring to a boil. Reduce the heat to low and simmer for about 25 minutes, until the yam is cooked through and can be pierced with a fork.

3. Transfer the soup to a high-powered blender and add the whole peeled lime, tahini, and sea salt. Blend until smooth.

4. To serve, divide the spinach among four bowls and ladle the soup on top. Garnish each serving with a sprinkle of chopped spinach, 1 tablespoon green onions, and 2 teaspoons sesame seeds.

Tichi's Gazpacho

CONTRIBUTED BY CHEF JOSÉ ANDRÉS

Serves: 4

Prep Time: 10 minutes
Cook Time: 30 minutes

Soup Base

1 cucumber, peeled, seeded, and chopped

1 green bell pepper, stemmed, seeded, and diced

3 pounds ripe plum tomatoes

2 cloves garlic, peeled

¼ cup sherry vinegar

½ cup Oloroso sherry

½ cup Spanish extra virgin olive oil

2 cups filtered water

Garnish

½ cucumber

½ green bell pepper

6 to 8 cherry tomatoes

¼ cup Spanish extra virgin olive oil

2 teaspoons sea salt

This delicious, easy-to-make gazpacho was shared by my friend José Andrés, chef and owner of ThinkFoodGroup and minibar. It's one of his favorite recipes from his wife, Tichi. I love the fresh, tangy taste of the chilled soup on a warm summer day when tomatoes are at their best. It makes an excellent appetizer or side dish, and it's bursting with vitamin C and antioxidants.

1. For the soup base: Combine the cucumber, bell pepper, tomatoes, garlic, vinegar, sherry, olive oil, and water in a food processor or blender. Purée until everything is well blended and smooth.

2. Strain the gazpacho through a medium strainer into a pitcher. Refrigerate for at least 30 minutes.

3. While the soup chills, prepare the garnish: Dice the cucumber and green bell pepper and halve the tomatoes.

4. To serve, distribute the cherry tomato halves, diced cucumber, and green peppers in each bowl and pour the gazpacho on top. Drizzle each bowl with olive oil, sprinkle with salt, and serve.

Thai Broccoli Fish Stew

Serves: 4

Prep Time: 15 minutes
Cook Time: 20 to
25 minutes

2 tablespoons avocado oil

1 large white onion, finely
diced (about 1½ cups)

½ cup tightly packed fresh
cilantro, finely chopped

¼ cup plus 2 tablespoons
red curry paste

2 teaspoons ume plum vinegar

1 tablespoon gluten-free
tamari

1 tablespoon pressed garlic

5 cups finely chopped broccoli

4 cups (32 ounces) vegetable
or chicken broth

1 can full-fat unsweetened
coconut milk

2 tablespoons lime juice

3 tablespoons gluten-free,
no-sugar-added fish sauce

10 ounces baby spinach

1 pound boneless, skinless
wild-caught salmon, cut into
1-inch cubes

½ cup minced green onions

⅓ cup minced fresh mint

1 lime, quartered

I just love the tangy, savory taste of coconut milk, ume vinegar, lime juice, and red curry in this savory salmon stew. It's the perfect base for poaching broccoli and hunks of fish until perfectly tender. The peppers in the red curry paste, along with ginger and garlic, are excellent for promoting circulation and increasing thermogenesis, which produces heat in the body and can even lead to a boost in fat burning.

1. Heat the avocado oil in a large pot over medium heat until shimmering. Add the onion and cook down for 5 minutes. Add the cilantro, curry paste, ume vinegar, and tamari, then stir well for 2 minutes. Add the garlic and broccoli and stir well so the broccoli is coated, then add the broth. Continue cooking over medium heat until the broccoli is tender, about 7 minutes. Stir in the coconut milk, lime juice, and fish sauce.

2. Completely submerge all the baby spinach in the soup, then add salmon and simmer until cooked through, 6 to 8 minutes, depending on the thickness of the fish.

3. Serve the soup right away, garnishing each portion with green onions, mint, and a lime wedge. If you need to make it ahead of time, wait to add the spinach and salmon until reheating.

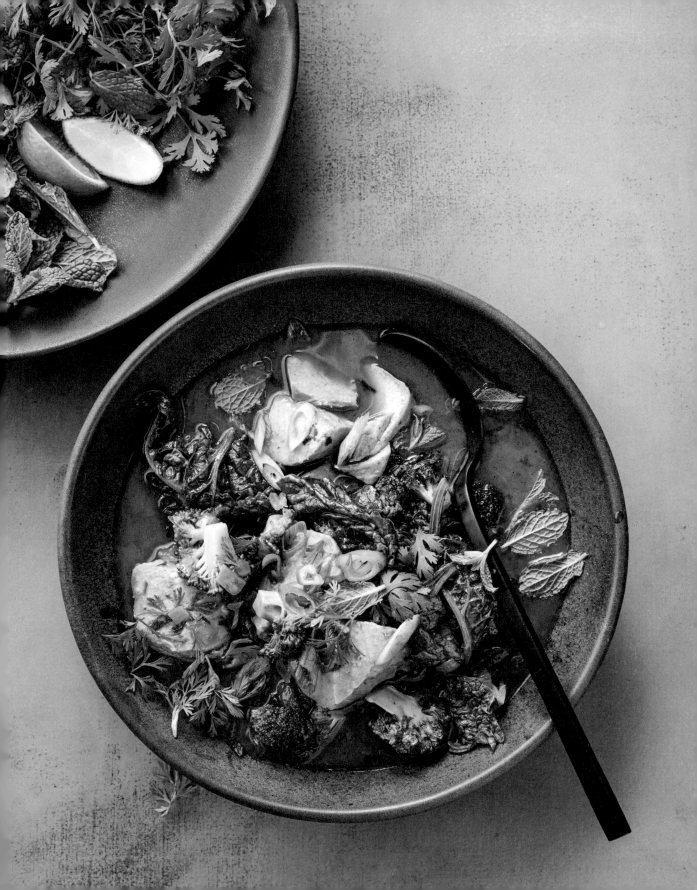

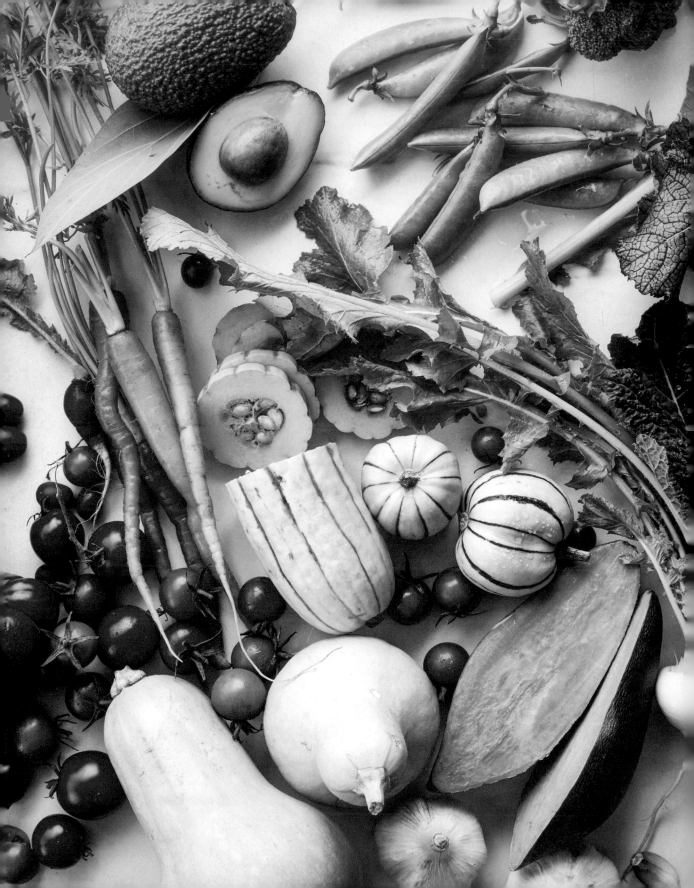

Sides

Complementing an entrée with delectable sides can take your meal to the next level. A side dish is a nice opportunily lo add more colorful veggies and nutrients to your plate; it's also a great way to please a variety of different palates. Many of these recipes can be enjoyed on their own as a snack, or you can combine several to make a complete tapas-style meal.

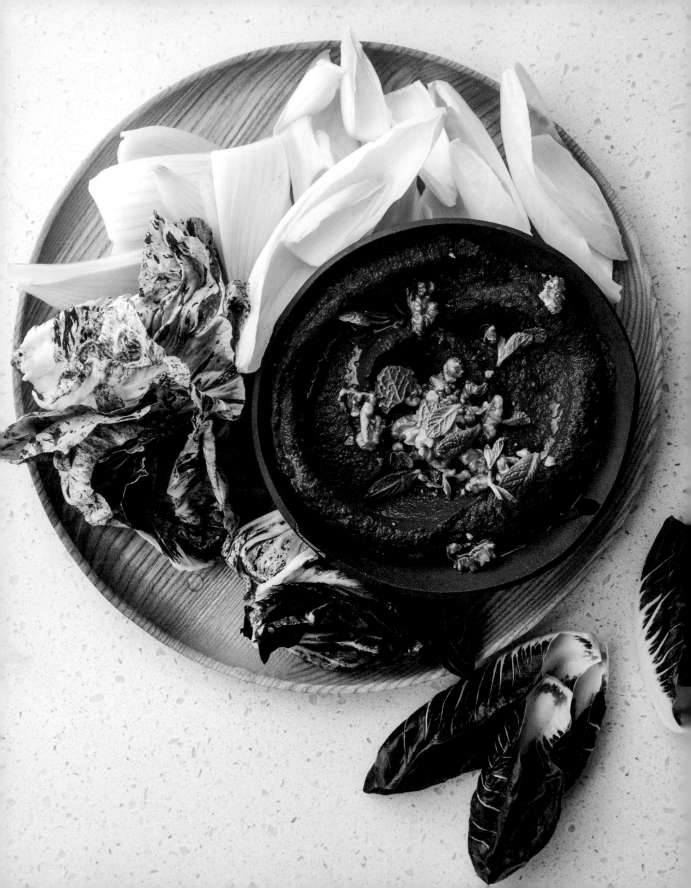

Blushing Beet Dip

Makes: 1 cup

Prep Time: 10 minutes

Cook Time: 1 hour

1 cup plus 1½ teaspoons sea salt

1 medium red beet

⅓ cup cold filtered water

¾ cup tahini

¼ cup lemon juice

2 cloves garlic, minced

6 raw walnuts, coarsely chopped

5 large mint leaves, torn

Drizzle of extra virgin olive oil (optional)

I always tell my patients to eat the rainbow so they can take advantage of all the powerful phytonutrients found in colorful plant foods. This richly colored dip is high in antioxidants from crimson beets, along with calcium from creamy tahini. It's a beautiful way to add extra color to your day; I love serving it with my Savory Seed Crackers (page 273) and a variety of leafy vegetables, like radicchio and endive.

1. Preheat the oven to 425°F.

2. Pour the 1 cup salt into a large pile on a baking sheet and create a well in the middle. Place the beet in the well of salt and sprinkle some of the salt on top. Roast until a paring knife can easily pierce the beet, about 1 hour. When the beet is cool enough to handle, peel the skin by rubbing with your hand, then roughly chop.

3. Combine the beet, water, tahini, lemon juice, garlic, and remaining 1½ teaspoons salt in a food processor and blend until smooth.

4. Transfer the dip to a bowl. Top with the walnuts, mint, and a drizzle of olive oil (if using).

Chermoula Cauliflower Steaks

Steak doesn't have to come from a cow—these cauliflower steaks are an amazing alternative, with a fresh chermoula sauce that takes them to the next level. Cauliflower is a great source of immune-boosting vitamins C and B₆, which help promote a good mood, healthy blood cells, and much more. This recipe makes extra chermoula. Save it in a jar in the fridge for up to a week and enjoy it as a quick dip for leftover cauliflower florets, or spoon it over eggs for an easy breakfast.

Serves: 4

Prep Time: 15 minutes
Cook Time: 25 minutes

Cauliflower Steaks

4 medium heads cauliflower

¼ cup plus 2 tablespoons avocado oil

3 tablespoons lemon juice

3 tablespoons capers, rinsed and minced

¾ teaspoon garlic powder

½ teaspoon paprika

¾ teaspoon sea salt

½ teaspoon freshly ground black pepper

Chermoula

¾ cup raw slivered almonds

2 cups finely chopped fresh parsley, plus more for garnish

1 cup loosely packed fresh cilantro, finely chopped, plus more for garnish

½ cup plus 1 tablespoon extra virgin olive oil

¼ cup lemon juice

2 tablespoons filtered water

1 tablespoon gluten-free tamari

3 tablespoons capers

1 tablespoon pressed garlic

1 tablespoon minced seeded jalapeño

½ teaspoon smoked paprika

¼ teaspoon chili flakes

½ teaspoon sea salt

1. Preheat the oven to 450°F.

2. For the steaks: Remove the green leaves and trim the stems from the cauliflower. Cut one head in half lengthwise through the center. Then cut a 1½-inch-thick steak from each half. Repeat with other cauliflower heads, for a total of eight steaks. You'll have lots of extra cauliflower florets and crumbles; save for a snack or use in another recipe. Arrange the steaks on two baking sheets.

3. Mix the avocado oil, lemon juice, capers, garlic powder, paprika, salt, and pepper in a bowl. Drizzle or brush half this mixture over the cauliflower steaks. Roast the cauliflower for 12 minutes. Flip the steaks, rotate the pans between top and bottom oven racks, and drizzle or brush with the remaining avocado oil mixture. Place back in the oven and roast for another 10 to 13 minutes, until the steaks are browned and the thickest part of a stem can be slightly pierced with a fork—it doesn't need to go all the way through.

4. For the chermoula: While the cauliflower roasts, toast the slivered almonds in a medium sauté pan over medium-high heat, stirring and shaking continuously, until fragrant and golden, about 5 minutes.

5. In a high-speed blender or food processor, mix ½ cup of the toasted almonds, the parsley, cilantro, olive oil, lemon juice, water, tamari, capers, garlic, jalapeño, paprika, chili flakes, and salt until a uniform sauce forms.

6. Serve the steaks on a platter, drizzled with the chermoula and sprinkled with the parsley, cilantro, and remaining slivered almonds.

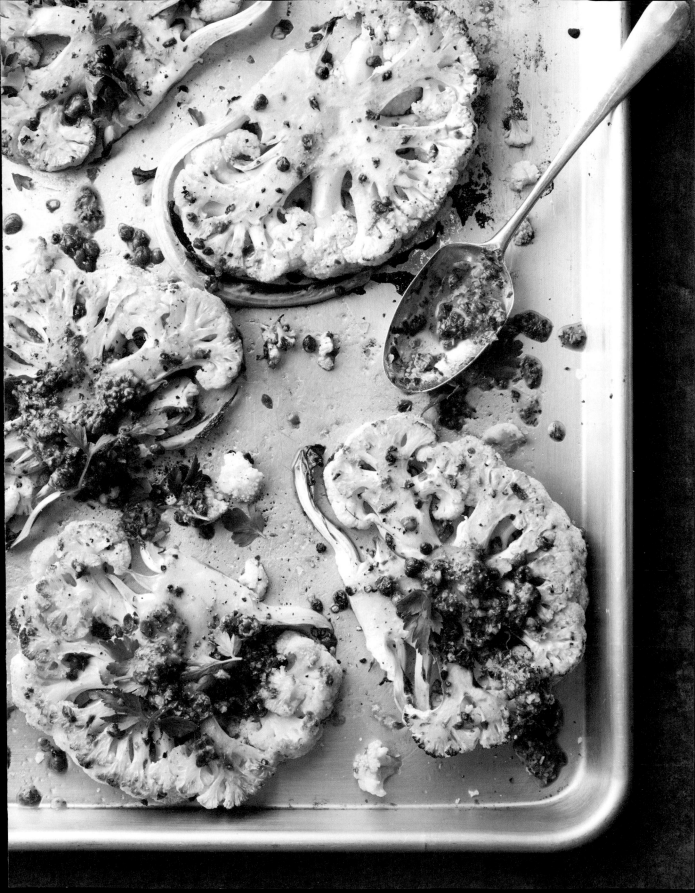

Coconut-Pecan Yam Bake

CONTRIBUTED BY DEANNA MINICH, MD

Serves: 4

Prep Time: 10 minutes
Cook Time: 1 hour

3 medium yams

1¼ cups light unsweetened coconut milk

1 tablespoon raw honey (optional, not vegan friendly)

4 tablespoons raw pecans, chopped

4 tablespoons unsweetened shredded coconut

¾ teaspoon ground nutmeg

½ teaspoon ground cinnamon

My friend Dr. Deanna Minich was kind enough to share this delectable recipe—it's a great example of her colorful approach to healthy cooking. When combined with creamy coconut milk, yams can be mashed into an incredibly smooth, antioxidant-rich side dish that makes the perfect vehicle for warm spices like cinnamon and nutmeg along with buttery pecans.

1. Preheat the oven to 350°F.

2. Place the yams on a baking sheet and bake for 1 hour, until soft. Let cool slightly.

3. When the yams are cool enough to handle comfortably, remove the skin, transfer the flesh to a large bowl, and break into small pieces using a fork. Pour in the coconut milk, stirring and mashing until the mixture is smooth.

4. Add honey (if using), 3 tablespoons of the pecans, 3 tablespoons of the coconut, and the nutmeg and cinnamon and mix well. Pour into a medium casserole dish. Sprinkle the top with the remaining 1 tablespoon each pecans and coconut. Serve either warm or cold.

Easy Sesame Super Greens

Serves: 4

Prep Time: 10 minutes
Cook Time: 5 minutes

Dressing

1 tablespoon micro-grated peeled fresh ginger

2 tablespoons toasted sesame oil

2 tablespoons gluten-free tamari

1 tablespoon lime juice

1 tablespoon almond butter

1½ teaspoons pressed garlic

Greens

1 small head broccoli, chopped into small florets (about 2 cups)

1 bunch asparagus, cut into 1-inch pieces (about 2 cups)

2 cups chopped baby bok choy

Garnish

1 tablespoon black sesame seeds

This recipe is proof that healthy eating does not have to take a lot of time! The beautiful variety of green veggies is a great source of folate and vitamin K, and tossing them in a creamy sauce of toasted sesame oil and almond butter with ginger, lime, and garlic creates a perfect balance of tangy and savory flavors.

1. For the dressing: Squeeze the grated ginger in your hands or twist in a piece of cheesecloth to release the juice into a small jar; discard the ginger pulp. Add the sesame oil, tamari, lime juice, almond butter, and garlic to the ginger juice and mix well. Set the dressing aside.

2. For the greens: Bring 1 inch water to a boil in a saucepan. Place the broccoli, asparagus, and bok choy in a steamer basket and place in the pot. Cover and steam for 5 minutes, stirring the vegetables once halfway through so they get equal access to the heat, until cooked through.

3. Carefully transfer the vegetables to a serving bowl, add the dressing and black sesame seeds, and toss.

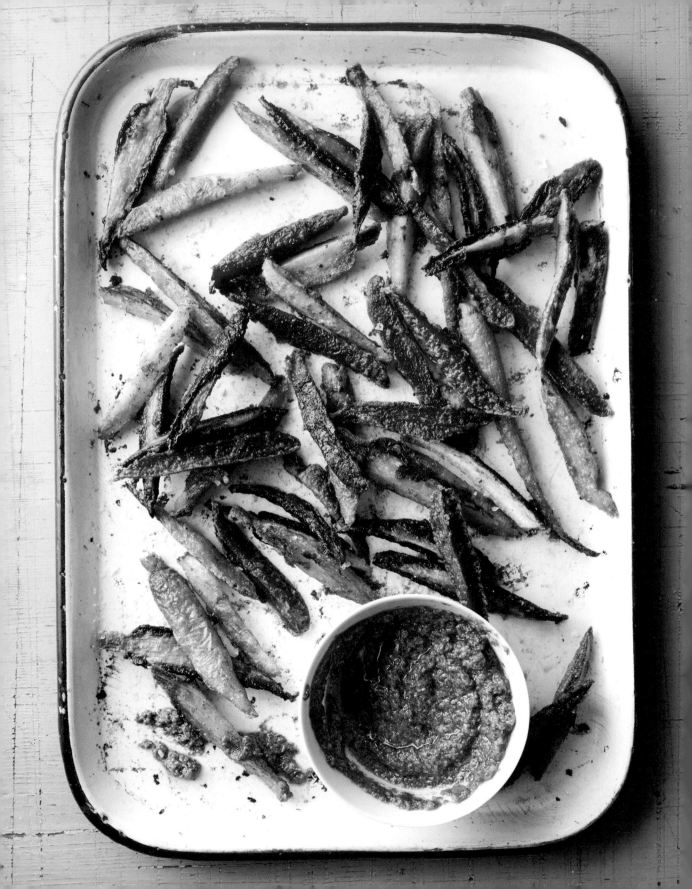

Crispy Carrot Fries with Pesto

Believe it or not, you can make delightfully crispy fries without any frying at all. A dusting of tapioca flour and spices creates a light, flavorful coating for these irresistible multicolored fries. To serve alongside, pine nuts, basil, and fresh lemon blend into a delicious, zesty, dairy-free pesto that is perfect for dipping. This dish is such a crowd pleaser you may want to double it!

Serves: 4

Prep Time: 10 minutes
Cook Time: 25 minutes

Carrot Fries

6 large rainbow carrots

2 tablespoons avocado oil

2 tablespoons tapioca flour

1 teaspoon garlic powder

½ teaspoon ground coriander

½ teaspoon ground sage

1 teaspoon sea salt

¼ teaspoon black pepper

Pesto

1 cup pine nuts

2 cups chopped fresh basil leaves

1 tablespoon pressed garlic

¼ cup extra virgin olive oil

1½ teaspoons grated lemon zest

2 tablespoons lemon juice

½ teaspoon onion powder

¼ teaspoon sea salt

½ teaspoon freshly grated black pepper

1. Preheat the oven to 425°F.

2. For the fries: Make sure the carrots are very dry before cutting into fries. Trim the tops and ends and cut each carrot lengthwise in half. Cut those pieces in half crosswise, then cut the wedges into thirds to create fry-size sticks. Toss the carrot fries with the avocado oil in a large bowl, using hands to thoroughly coat.

3. In a small bowl, combine the tapioca flour, garlic powder, coriander, sage, salt, and pepper and stir well. Pour the tapioca mixture over carrots and use hands to toss thoroughly until all the flour has been absorbed by the oil.

4. Arrange the carrots on two baking sheets, making sure they are evenly spaced and not touching at all. Bake for 12 minutes. Flip the fries, rotate the pans between the top and bottom racks of the oven. Bake for another 12 to 15 minutes, until the fries are lightly browned and crispy.

5. For the pesto: While the fries bake, toast the pine nuts: Heat a medium sauté pan over medium-high heat. Add the pine nuts and toast, stirring frequently, until fragrant and golden, about 3 minutes. Remove from the heat.

6. Combine the pine nuts, basil, garlic, olive oil, lemon zest and juice, onion powder, salt, and pepper in a food processor and blend well.

7. Serve the carrot fries fresh out of the oven with the pesto for dipping.

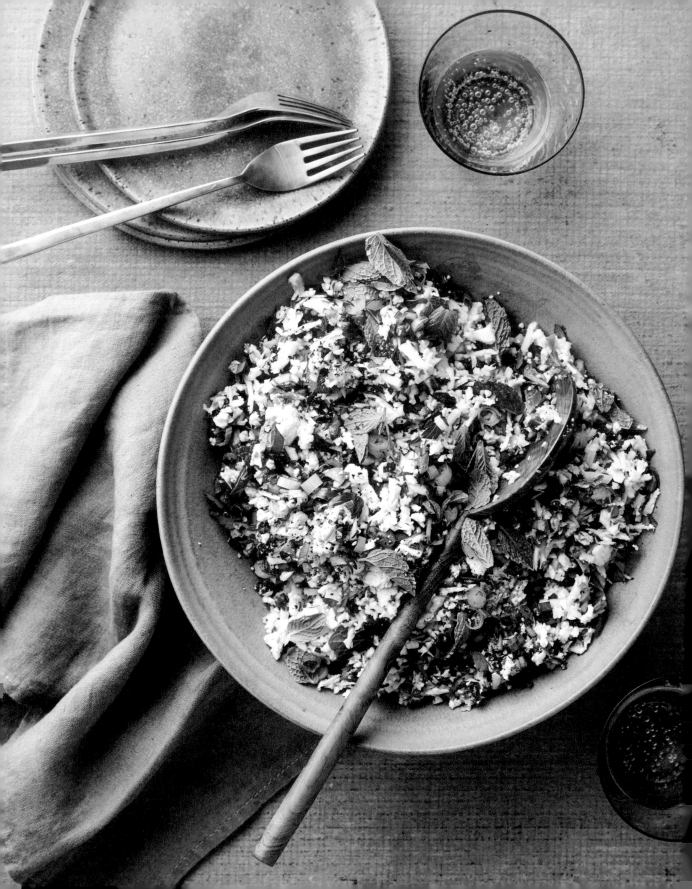

Grain-Free Cauliflower Tabbouleh

Serves: 4

Prep Time: 15 minutes

1 large head cauliflower

1 cup fresh parsley leaves, minced

½ cup sundried tomatoes, minced

⅓ cup capers, minced

1 tablespoon pressed garlic

2 tablespoons plus 1 teaspoon lemon juice, plus more for seasoning

¼ teaspoon ground cumin

¼ teaspoon sea salt, plus more for seasoning

¼ teaspoon black pepper, plus more for seasoning

¼ cup extra virgin olive oil

½ cup fresh mint leaves, minced

⅓ cup minced green onions

½ cup Castelvetrano olives, pitted and minced (optional)

I love having a big batch of this tabbouleh on hand throughout the week. Traditional tabbouleh is made with bulgur wheat, but I swapped that out for finely chopped cauliflower to make this recipe gluten- and grain-free. Just use a food processor to rice your cauliflower and you'll be amazed at how quick and easy this ultra-flavorful recipe is to make. Leftovers will last in the fridge for up to 3 days and are especially delicious wrapped in seaweed with a little smoked salmon.

1. To rice the cauliflower, remove the outer green leaves and most of the stem and chop the remaining cauliflower into medium chunks. Pulse in a food processor until the cauliflower resembles fine grains. Alternatively, you can grate the cauliflower on the large holes of a box grater.

2. Blend the parsley, sundried tomatoes, capers, garlic, lemon juice, cumin, salt, and pepper in a small food processor until combined into a chunky paste.

3. Add the parsley mixture to the riced cauliflower and stir well. Add the olive oil, mint, green onions, and olives (if using) and toss together. Add more lemon, salt, or pepper to taste.

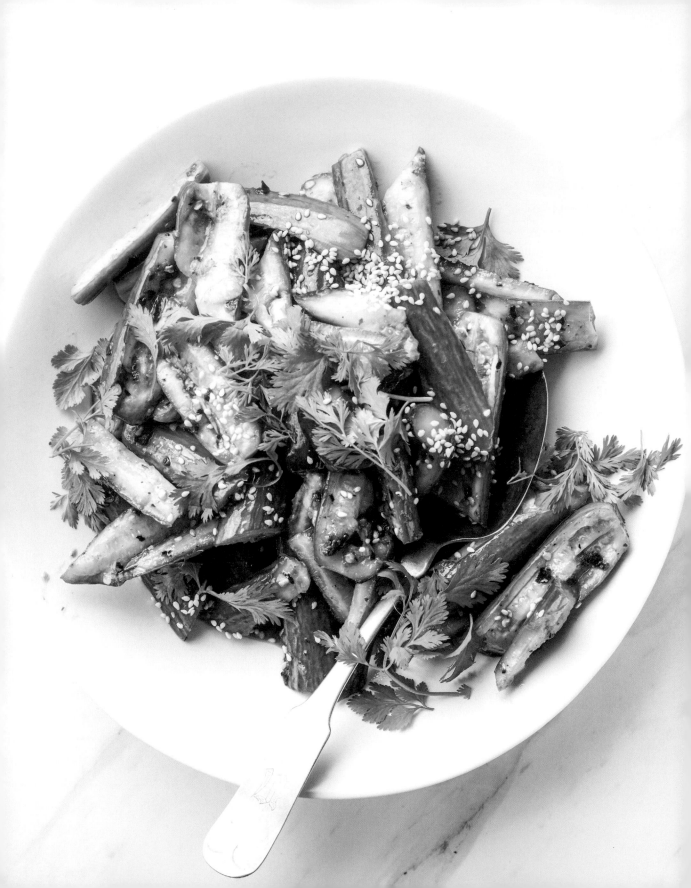

Smashed Persian Cucumbers

Serves: 4 to 6

Prep Time: 10 minutes,
plus 30 minutes standing

2 pounds Persian cucumbers

2 teaspoons pink Himalayan
salt or sea salt

2 teaspoons coconut sugar
(optional)

2 large cloves garlic, minced

2½ tablespoons coconut
aminos

2 tablespoons sesame oil

1½ tablespoons rice vinegar

1 tablespoon extra virgin
olive oil

2 teaspoons chili flakes
(optional)

¼ cup loosely packed fresh
cilantro leaves

Toasted white sesame seeds

Simple food can be the most delicious. This fun smashing technique takes cucumbers to a whole new level, creating a tender texture that soaks up the amazing flavors of sesame, garlic, and chili flakes. It's crisp and fresh and makes an excellent side dish for a wide variety of entrées, like my Seared Scallops with Avocado-Yuzu Sauce (page 177).

1. Cut the cucumbers crosswise into 4-inch pieces. Stand one piece on a flat surface. Lay the blade of a large knife flat on top, and smash down gently, then tear into smaller pieces at the natural breaking points. Repeat to smash all the cucumber pieces.

2. Place the cucumber pieces in a strainer and toss with 1 teaspoon of the salt and 1 teaspoon of the coconut sugar (if using). Place a bowl on top of the cucumbers with something that can serve as a weight inside it. Let drain for at least 30 minutes. Use paper towels to pat the cucumbers dry and place in a bowl.

3. In a small bowl, combine the remaining 1 teaspoon salt and 1 teaspoon sugar (if using) with the garlic, coconut aminos, sesame oil, vinegar, olive oil, and chili flakes, then pour over the cucumbers and toss. Serve with whole cilantro leaves and sesame seeds sprinkled on top.

Zesty Sautéed Summer Squash

Serves: 4

Prep Time: 10 minutes
Cook Time: 15 minutes

3 tablespoons avocado oil

1 large zucchini, sliced into rounds

1 large yellow squash, sliced into rounds

1 yellow onion, thinly sliced

½ large green chile (mild or spicy), seeded and sliced into rounds

3 cloves garlic, minced

½ teaspoon sea salt

¼ teaspoon freshly ground black pepper

6 fresh mint leaves, torn

6 fresh basil leaves, torn

Grated zest of 1 lemon

I love how easy this recipe is—it's a great weeknight staple that helps you get vegetables on the table in no time at all. Garlic and onions both have immune-boosting properties, so they team up perfectly with the squash, which is loaded with vitamin C. Lemon zest and herbs add an extra layer of bright, fresh flavor.

1. Heat 2 tablespoons of avocado oil in a large cast-iron pan over high heat until shimmering. Add the squash and cook until tender, about 4 minutes. Remove the squash from the pan and set aside.

2. Heat the remaining 1 tablespoon avocado oil in the same pan over medium heat. Add the onion and chile and cook until the onion is golden brown, about 5 minutes. Add the garlic, salt, and pepper and keep stirring for 2 minutes.

3. Return the squash to the pan, stir, and cook everything together for another 2 minutes, until warm throughout. Remove the pan from the heat and allow to cool for several minutes, then garnish with the mint, basil, and lemon zest.

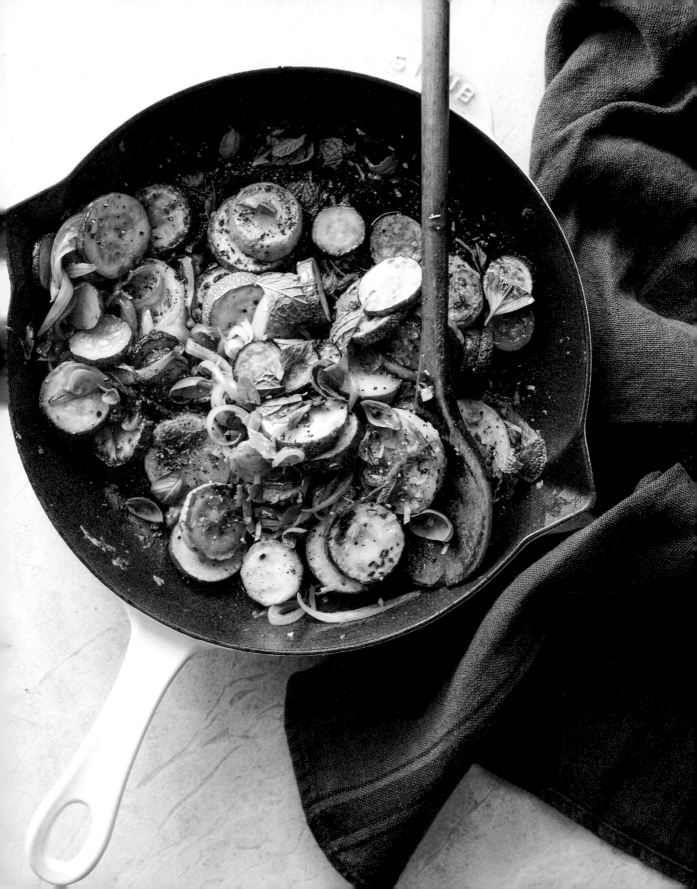

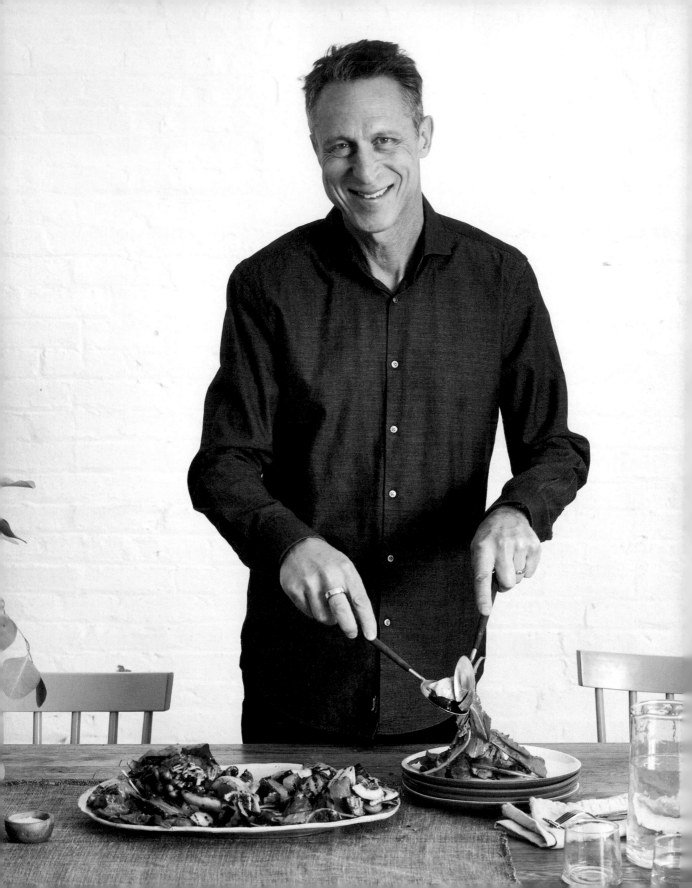

Entrées

The main course! There is always much excitement around this star of the show, and rightly so. No matter your protein preference—poultry, red meat, seafood, or totally plant-based—I've got you covered with an amazing variety of show-stopping entrées. I love combining different colors, flavors, and textures all on one plate to create a beautiful, satisfying, and nutritious dinner. Many of these recipes work as complete meals on their own, but you can always incorporate any of my soups, salads, or sides for a more diverse menu.

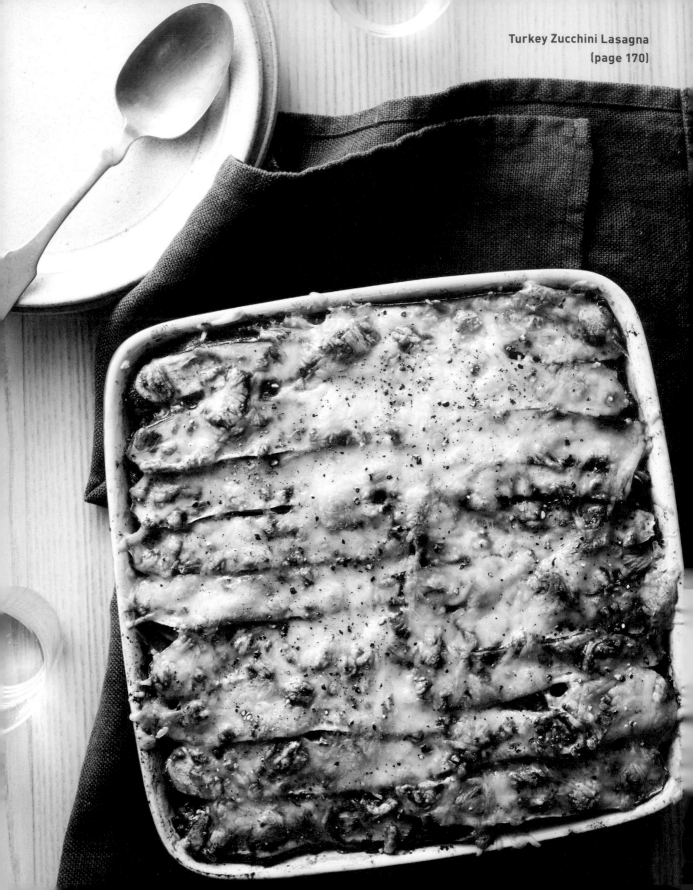

Turkey Zucchini Lasagna
(page 170)

Poultry

Say goodbye to boring, dry chicken and hello to a variety of juicy, flavorful poultry options that you can incorporate into your weekly meal plan. From skewered breasts to slow-cooked thighs, these mouthwatering recipes will add plenty of protein and beneficial nutrients to your plate. When shopping, choose pasture-raised poultry for the cleanest possible cuts.

Almond Chicken Skewers with Green Beans

Serves: 4

Prep Time: 15 minutes, plus 30 minutes marinating

Cook Time: 25 minutes

Chicken and Marinade

½ cup light unsweetened coconut milk

3 tablespoons lime juice

1 teaspoon curry powder

1 teaspoon garlic powder

¼ teaspoon sea salt

1½ pounds pasture-raised chicken breasts, cut into 1-inch strips

Green Beans

1 pound (4 cups) green beans

1 tablespoon avocado oil

¼ cup finely chopped shallots

1 tablespoon filtered water

Almond Sauce

½ cup almond butter

½ cup light unsweetened coconut milk

2 tablespoons tightly packed minced fresh cilantro

2 tablespoons lime juice

2 tablespoons gluten-free tamari

2 teaspoons pressed garlic

1 teaspoon curry powder

¼ teaspoon cayenne

This meal is sure to become a new family favorite—rich coconut milk, tangy lime juice, and a hint of spice from curry powder create an amazing marinade for tender grilled chicken skewers that are drizzled with a creamy Thai-inspired almond butter sauce. Green beans add a welcome addition of color, crunch, and fiber, and are high in the mineral silicon, which encourages healthier connective tissues and bones.

1. For the chicken and marinade: Mix the coconut milk, lime juice, curry powder, garlic powder, and sea salt in a shallow dish. Add the chicken and marinate in the fridge for 30 minutes. At the same time, soak 8 bamboo skewers in water.

2. For the green beans: Cut the hard ends off the beans, then cut in half. Heat the avocado oil in a small sauté pan over medium-low heat until shimmering. Add the shallots and cook until translucent, about 5 minutes. Add the green beans and cook for 8 minutes. Turn the heat to medium, add the water, and stir well. Cook until the beans are tender, about 2 minutes longer. Remove from the heat.

3. For the sauce: Blend the almond butter, coconut milk, cilantro, lime juice, tamari, garlic, curry powder, and cayenne in a high-speed blender or mini food processor until creamy.

4. To toast the almonds for the garnish: Cook in a dry medium sauté pan over medium-high heat, stirring frequently, until fragrant and toasted, about 5 minutes.

5. When the chicken is almost done marinating, heat a grill or grill pan to medium-high.

Garnish

¼ cup slivered almonds, toasted

2 tablespoons chopped fresh cilantro

6. Thread the chicken onto the skewers. Grill 4 minutes per side, or until completely cooked through with an internal temperature of 165°F. (Alternatively, you can bake the skewered chicken on a parchment-lined baking sheet in a 375°F oven for 25 minutes, until 165°F internal temperature.)

7. To serve, divide the green beans among four plates and top with the chicken skewers. Drizzle generously with sauce and garnish with cilantro and toasted almonds.

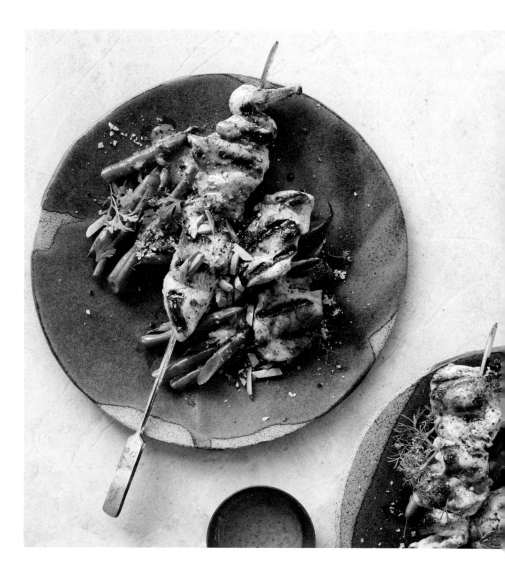

Serves: 4

Prep Time: 15 minutes
Cook Time: 25 minutes

Meatballs

1 cup loosely packed fresh cilantro, finely chopped

¼ cup loosely packed fresh mint, finely chopped

¼ cup loosely packed, finely chopped green onions

1 tablespoon minced seeded jalapeño

1 tablespoon onion powder

2 teaspoons micro-grated peeled fresh ginger

½ teaspoon grated lemon zest (optional)

¾ teaspoon sea salt

1 pound pasture-raised ground turkey (90 percent lean or less)

1 large pasture-raised egg

2 tablespoons almond meal

Noodles

4 cups spiralized butternut squash noodles

2 tablespoons avocado oil

¼ teaspoon sea salt

¼ teaspoon freshly ground black pepper

Juice of ½ large lemon

Garnish

Extra virgin olive oil, for drizzling

½ cup fresh basil leaves, torn

Coarse sea salt

Herbed Mini Meatballs with Butternut Noodles

Green onions and fresh mint and cilantro provide herbaceous flavor and medicinal benefits (including antioxidant and antibacterial properties) to these little meatballs. Pile them on my easy-to-make lemony butternut noodles for a comforting yet nourishing meal any night of the week.

1. Preheat the oven to 400°F; line two baking sheets with parchment paper.

2. For the meatballs: In a large mixing bowl, thoroughly combine the cilantro, mint, green onions, jalapeño, onion powder, ginger, lemon zest (if using), and salt. Using hands, gently toss the turkey with the herb mixture. Whisk the egg in a small bowl, then add the almond meal and mix well. Using your fingers like a pitchfork, gently work the egg and almond mixture into the turkey, taking care not to overmix.

3. Use hands to roll 1-tablespoon portions of the mixture into meatballs. Place on one baking sheet, evenly spaced. Bake for 12 minutes, flip the meatballs, then bake for another 12 to 14 minutes, until golden brown.

4. For the noodles: While the meatballs bake, place the butternut noodles on the other baking sheet, drizzle with the avocado oil, and sprinkle with the salt and pepper. Toss together, then roast for 10 to 15 minutes, until tender. Remove from the oven and toss with the lemon juice.

5. Divide the noodles among four plates and top with the meatballs, a drizzle of olive oil, and the fresh basil. Add coarse sea salt to taste.

Slow-Cooked Chicken Thighs with Kale

Serves: 6

Prep Time: 20 minutes
Cook Time: 6 hours

6 pasture-raised boneless, skinless chicken thighs (about 1½ pounds)

1 teaspoon paprika

1 teaspoon sea salt

¼ teaspoon freshly ground black pepper

2 teaspoons avocado oil

1 (15.5-ounce) can cannellini beans

1 large yellow onion, finely chopped (about 2 cups)

1 carrot, thinly sliced into rounds (about 1 cup)

1 cup vegetable broth

Grated zest of 1 lemon

2 tablespoons lemon juice

1 tablespoon balsamic vinegar

2 tablespoons capers, rinsed and minced

1 tablespoon pressed garlic

2 sprigs fresh thyme

1½ teaspoons dried basil

1½ teaspoons dried oregano

10 Castelvetrano olives, pitted and chopped

1 bunch green curly kale, deveined and finely chopped (4 cups tightly packed)

¼ cup chopped fresh cilantro

I love using my slow cooker to make warm, satisfying, one-bowl meals. You can just throw everything in, set it, and forget it—then a few hours later you have a delicious dinner ready and waiting. This dish covers all your bases: high-quality fat and protein from pastured chicken, folate and phytonutrients from curly kale, and fiber and slow-burning carbs from cannellini beans.

1. Season the chicken with the paprika, salt, and pepper. Heat the avocado oil in a large sauté pan over medium-high heat until shimmering. Add the chicken and sear on each side for about 3 minutes, until browned.

2. Transfer the chicken to the slow cooker and add the beans, onion, carrot, broth, lemon zest and juice, vinegar, capers, garlic, thyme, basil, and oregano. Stir well, cover, and cook on low for 5 hours and 50 minutes.

3. Add the olives and kale, stir, and cook for 10 minutes longer.

4. When ready to serve, divide the chicken, beans, and vegetables among six bowls and top each serving with fresh cilantro.

Turkey Zucchini Lasagna

Serves: 6 to 8

Prep Time: 1 hour
Cook Time: 25 minutes

Zucchini Noodles

9 medium zucchini

½ teaspoon sea salt

Chard

2 tablespoons avocado oil

1 tablespoon plus 1 teaspoon pressed garlic

1 teaspoon sea salt

2 bunches Swiss or rainbow chard, deveined and cut into thin strips

1 tablespoon lemon juice

Turkey Filling

1½ tablespoons avocado oil

2 teaspoons minced seeded jalapeño (optional)

2 teaspoons pressed garlic

2 teaspoons chili powder

1 teaspoon smoked paprika

1 teaspoon dried oregano

1 teaspoon onion powder

1½ pounds pasture-raised ground turkey

1½ cups no-sugar-added marinara sauce

1 cup fresh basil leaves, chopped

1¼ teaspoons sea salt

Zucchini noodles are an excellent replacement for lasagna noodles since they don't have refined flour and gluten. With layers of tangy tomato-based turkey filling and nutrient-dense Swiss chard, this is a delicious yet ultra-healthy lasagna that is sure to please everyone. I love having the leftovers for lunch. It will keep covered in the fridge for up to 3 days.

1. Preheat the oven to 375°F; line two baking sheets with parchment paper.

2. For the zucchini noodles: Cut the ends off the zucchini and thinly slice into longitudinal strips, like lasagna noodles, about ¼-inch thick. Use a mandoline if you have one to ensure consistent thickness. You want 22 strips. Evenly arrange the strips on the two lined baking sheets, then sprinkle evenly with the salt. Bake for 5 minutes. Rotate the pans between the top and bottom oven racks and bake for another 5 minutes, until tender.

3. For the chard: Heat the avocado oil in a large sauté pan over medium heat until shimmering. Add the garlic and salt and cook for 30 seconds, stirring well. Add the chard in batches, stirring well to spread the greens evenly around the pan. Once all the greens are wilted, after 2 to 3 minutes, reduce the heat to low and add the lemon juice. Transfer the chard to a colander to drain.

4. For the filling: Heat the avocado oil in a sauté pan over medium-low heat. When the oil is warm, add the jalapeño, garlic, chili powder, paprika, oregano, and onion powder. Sauté this spice mixture for 2 minutes. Increase the heat to medium, add the turkey, and cook for 8 minutes, stirring constantly. Add the marinara sauce and basil and cook for 2 minutes. Add the salt, stir well, and remove from the heat.

6 ounces goat's milk Cheddar cheese, finely grated (about 1½ cups)

1 teaspoon freshly cracked black pepper

Garnish

¼ cup thinly sliced fresh basil

5. Assemble the lasagna by arranging a layer of zucchini strips on the bottom of an 8x8-inch baking dish, then cover with half the turkey filling. Add another layer of zucchini, followed by all the chard, then ½ cup of the Cheddar. Repeat with the zucchini, the remaining meat, and the remaining 1 cup Cheddar spread evenly over the top. Sprinkle with fresh cracked pepper.

6. Bake for 25 minutes, until the sauce is bubbly and the cheese is melted. Let cool for several minutes before cutting. Top with thinly sliced basil and enjoy!

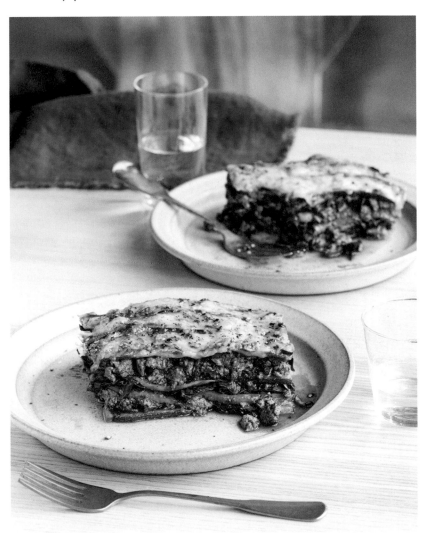

Wild Rice–Stuffed Chicken

There's something so classically beautiful (and delicious) about a whole roasted chicken. Thyme and sage give this bird a taste of the holidays, while the wild rice acts as both a savory stuffing and a nutty bed under the chicken to soak up all the savory spices. I love making this chicken for a big dinner with friends and family.

Chicken and Marinade

1 (3½-pound) pasture-raised whole chicken

¼ cup avocado oil

2 cloves garlic, minced

2 tablespoons tightly packed chopped fresh thyme

1 tablespoon tightly packed chopped fresh sage

Grated zest of 1 lemon

1½ teaspoons sea salt

1½ teaspoons freshly ground black pepper

Wild Rice Stuffing

1 cup wild rice

1½ teaspoons sea salt

3 tablespoons ghee or coconut oil

2¼ cups hot water

6 celery stalks, finely chopped

2 leeks, white parts only, finely chopped

2 large shallots, finely chopped

1 fennel bulb, cored and finely chopped

5 cloves garlic, minced

3 cremini mushrooms, sliced

2 tomatoes, seeded and diced

1 small zucchini, finely chopped

1. Preheat the oven to 375°F.

2. For the chicken: Rinse the chicken with cold water and pat dry. In a large bowl, combine all the marinade ingredients, add the chicken, and massage well. Place the bowl in the fridge while you make the stuffing.

3. For the stuffing: Rinse the wild rice and place in a small saucepan with the salt and 1 tablespoon of the ghee. Heat over high heat and stir until the ghee is melted. Add the hot water and bring to a boil. Reduce the heat, cover with a lid, and simmer for 30 to 35 minutes, until tender. Remove from the heat and keep covered for 10 minutes.

4. Meanwhile, in a large sauté pan over medium heat, melt the remaining 2 tablespoons ghee until shimmering. Add the celery, leeks, shallots, and fennel and cook for 10 to 15 minutes, until soft. Add the garlic and mushrooms and cook for 10 minutes. Add the tomatoes and stir for 5 minutes. Add the zucchini, thyme, sage, pepper, paprika, and chili flakes (if using) and cook for another 5 minutes. Remove the pan from the heat and add the chestnuts (if using), olives, and lemon zest. In a large bowl, mix the rice and veggies together.

5. Line the bottom of a Dutch oven with parchment paper. Add three-quarters of the stuffing to create a base, then stuff the chicken with the remaining stuffing. Place the stuffed chicken in the Dutch oven and drizzle the remaining oil and spices from the marinade bowl over the chicken. Tie the legs together with kitchen twine.

6. Cover the pot and roast the chicken for 1 hour. Uncover and roast for an additional 35 minutes, until a meat thermometer inserted near the inner thigh (be careful not to touch the bone) reads 165°F.

7. To serve, scoop rice from the bottom of the Dutch oven onto a platter and place the chicken on top.

2 tablespoons chopped
fresh thyme

2 tablespoons chopped
fresh sage

1 tablespoon freshly ground
black pepper

1 tablespoon smoked paprika

1 teaspoon chili flakes
(optional)

5 ounces roasted chestnuts,
peeled and chopped (optional)

1 cup Castelvetrano olives,
pitted and chopped

Grated zest of 1 lemon

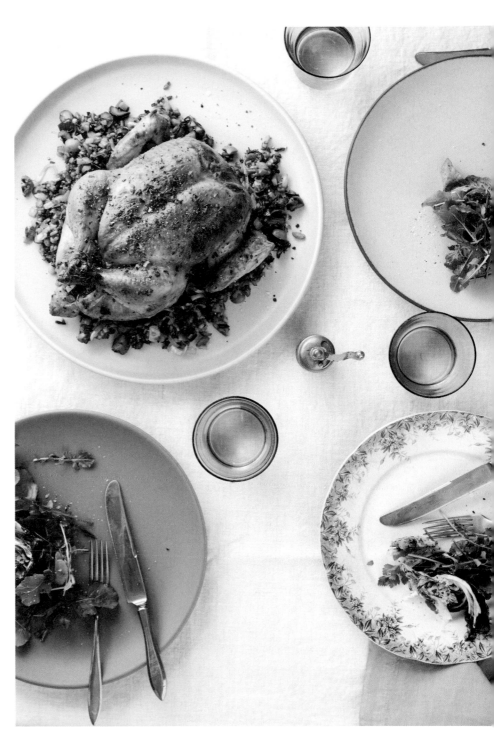

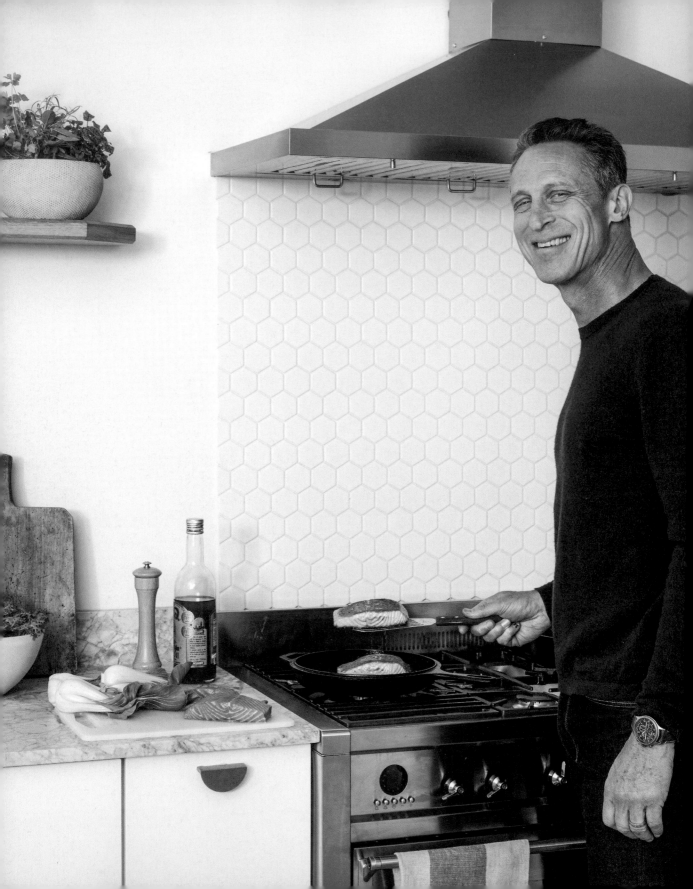

Seafood

Packed with nutrients like iodine, selenium, vitamin D, and omega-3 fatty acids, seafood is a nutritious and tasty protein that shines in a variety of cuisines. Scallops, salmon, and even sardines: This section has something from the sea for everyone. Opt for wild-caught, low-mercury, sustainably raised varieties to safely enjoy seafood as part of a healthy diet.

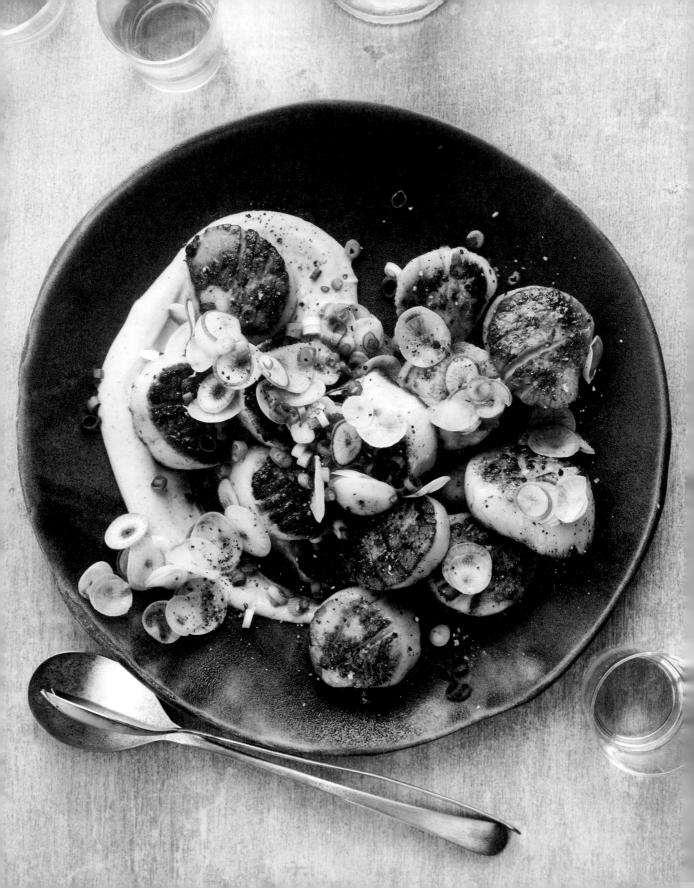

Seared Scallops with Avocado-Yuzu Sauce

Serves: 4

Prep Time: 10 minutes
Cook Time: 5 minutes

Avocado-Yuzu Sauce

2 medium avocados

¼ cup canned coconut cream
(unshaken so cream and water
are separated)

¼ cup plus 1 tablespoon
yuzu juice

3 tablespoons extra virgin
olive oil

1½ teaspoons toasted
sesame oil

¼ jalapeño, seeded (optional)

1 medium clove garlic, peeled

2 teaspoons sea salt

1 teaspoon freshly ground
black pepper

Scallops

12 large sea scallops

Pinch of sea salt

Pinch of freshly ground
black pepper

1 tablespoon avocado oil

Garnish

10 radishes, different colors,
thinly sliced into rounds

1 bunch green onions, sliced

This stunning dish is surprisingly easy to make. Yuzu, a citrus fruit with a bright, tangy taste, is often used in Japanese, Korean, and Chinese cooking. You can find fresh yuzu fruit or juice at many natural foods markets and specialty stores. Combined with rich avocado and coconut cream, it creates a delicious sauce for perfectly seared scallops. I love to serve the scallops with my Smashed Persian Cucumbers (page 159).

1. For the sauce: Combine all the ingredients in a blender and blend until smooth and creamy.

2. For the scallops: Pat the scallops dry and sprinkle with the salt and pepper. Heat the avocado oil in a large sauté pan over high heat. Once hot, add the scallops and cook for 2 minutes, then flip. Cook for another 2 to 3 minutes, until golden brown. Transfer to a paper towel.

3. To serve, spread the sauce on a platter and place the scallops on top. Garnish with thinly sliced radishes and green onions.

Coriander Salmon with Coconut-Tomato Salsa

Serves: 4

Prep Time: 20 minutes
Cook Time: 20 minutes

Coconut-Tomato Salsa

1 large tomato, roughly chopped

¼ cup diced red onion

¼ cup loosely packed fresh basil leaves, thinly sliced

2 tablespoons toasted unsweetened shredded coconut

2 tablespoons extra virgin olive oil

Juice of 1 lime

¼ teaspoon cayenne pepper

Salmon and Cauliflower

4 (4-ounce) wild-caught salmon fillets

2 tablespoons plus 2 teaspoons ghee or avocado oil

2 tablespoons ground coriander

2 teaspoons sea salt

1 small head cauliflower, leaves trimmed

1 red or orange bell pepper, stemmed, seeded, and sliced

10 asparagus spears, woody ends removed, cut into thirds

Ground coriander is actually the seed of the cilantro plant, and its warm, citrusy flavor makes it one of my favorite spices. It has been used medicinally for ages to support blood flow and calm the digestive system. Lime juice, basil leaves, coriander, and toasted coconut give the cauliflower rice and flaky salmon a fresh, tropical flare.

1. Preheat the oven to 350°F.

2. For the salsa: Combine all the ingredients in a medium bowl and stir well to combine; set aside. The salsa can be made up to one day in advance.

3. For the salmon: Place the salmon fillets in a baking dish, skin side down, and coat with 2 teaspoons of the ghee, the coriander, and 1 teaspoon of the salt. Bake for 10 to 12 minutes, until flaky and opaque.

4. For the cauliflower: Using a paring knife, cut the cauliflower florets away from the core; discard the core. Cut the florets into even smaller pieces, then pulse in a food processor in 3-second increments, until broken up into small ¼- to ½-inch pieces.

5. In a large skillet over medium heat, warm the remaining 2 tablespoons ghee until melted and shimmering. Add the cauliflower, bell pepper, and asparagus, stirring well to combine. Continue to cook, stirring occasionally, for 5 to 6 minutes, until the asparagus is just fork tender. Season with the remaining 1 teaspoon salt.

6. Divide the cauliflower mixture among four plates and top with the salmon fillets. Scoop some of the salsa over each piece of fish and serve.

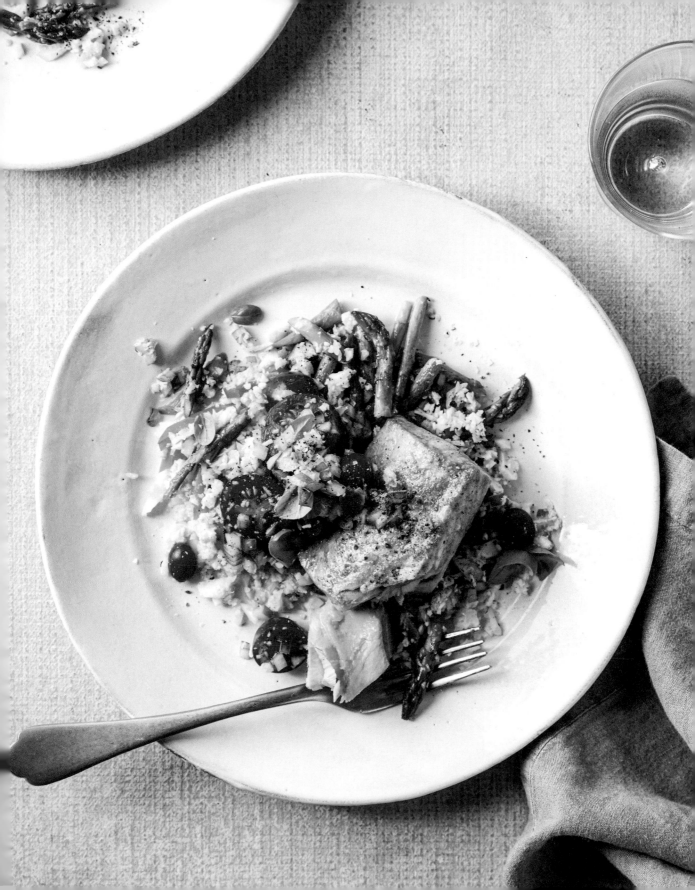

Herbed Sardine Cakes
with Avocado-Broccoli Salad

Serves: 4

Prep Time: 15 minutes, plus 30 minutes chilling

Cook Time: 45 minutes

Sardine Cakes

3 (4.4-ounce) cans wild-caught sardines in water, drained

⅓ cup finely diced white onion

¼ cup tightly packed fresh basil leaves, finely chopped

¼ cup tightly packed fresh cilantro leaves, finely chopped

3 tablespoons finely chopped green onions

1 tablespoon micro-grated peeled fresh ginger

2 teaspoons Dijon mustard

½ teaspoon apple cider vinegar

¼ teaspoon smoked paprika

1 teaspoon sea salt

¼ teaspoon freshly ground black pepper

2 large pasture-raised eggs, beaten

¾ cup almond flour

1 tablespoon avocado oil

Sardines are one of the healthiest fish, thanks to their high calcium and omega-3 content, and because they don't have the toxic burden that other types of seafood can carry. These sardine cakes are bursting with flavor from ginger, cilantro, and green onion, and they pair perfectly with the nutrient-dense broccoli salad.

1. For the sardine cakes: Mash the sardines with a fork in a large mixing bowl. Add the white onion, basil, cilantro, green onions, ginger, mustard, vinegar, paprika, salt, and pepper and mix well. Add the beaten eggs and almond flour and mix together. Shape into 8 patties. Place on a parchment-lined plate, cover, and refrigerate for at least 30 minutes.

2. Preheat the oven to 375°F. Line two baking sheets with parchment paper and grease with the avocado oil.

3. For the broccoli: Toss the broccoli with the lemon juice and garlic powder. Let sit for 10 minutes.

4. Place the fish cakes on one of the oiled sheets, evenly spaced. Pour the broccoli on the other prepared baking sheet, making sure each floret has space. Bake the fish cakes on the top rack of the oven for 20 minutes. Flip the cakes, move the pan to the bottom rack, and put the broccoli pan on the top rack. Bake both for 20 to 25 minutes, until the cakes are golden brown and the broccoli can be pierced easily with a fork.

Avocado-Broccoli Salad

2 large heads broccoli,
chopped into small florets
(6 heaping cups)

¼ cup lemon juice

1 tablespoon garlic powder

¼ cup tightly packed fresh
cilantro, chopped

3 tablespoons chopped
green onion

3 tablespoons toasted
sesame oil

2 teaspoons ume plum vinegar

1 teaspoon Dijon mustard

1 teaspoon raw honey
(optional)

1 teaspoon freshly ground
black pepper

2 avocados, pitted, peeled,
and chopped

1 tablespoon black sesame
seeds

5. While the fish cakes and broccoli are baking, make the dressing: In a large bowl, mix the cilantro, green onions, sesame oil, ume vinegar, mustard, honey (if using), and pepper. Add the chopped avocado and sesame seeds and stir gently to coat.

6. Add the broccoli to the dressing and toss. Divide the salad among four plates, add two sardine cakes on each plate alongside the salad, and serve.

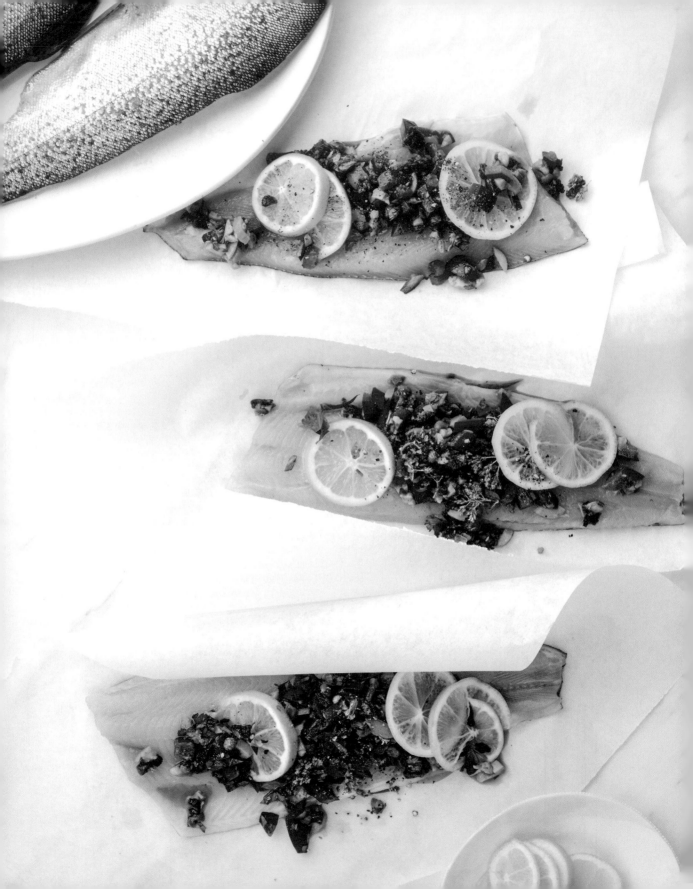

Mediterranean Trout en Papillote

Serves: 4

Prep Time: 15 minutes
Cook Time: 15 minutes

1 small red bell pepper, stemmed, seeded, and finely diced (about 1 cup)

½ cup sundried tomatoes, finely chopped

4 to 6 large Cerignola olives (or another type of green olive), pitted and chopped

2 tablespoons tightly packed minced fresh parsley

2 tablespoons avocado oil

1 tablespoon plus 1 teaspoon capers, rinsed and minced

1 teaspoon pressed garlic

1 teaspoon grated lemon zest

1 teaspoon dried oregano

1 teaspoon onion powder

½ teaspoon chili flakes (optional)

½ teaspoon freshly ground black pepper

4 (4-ounce) skin-on trout fillets

8 to 12 thin slices lemon

Sea salt

The classic French technique of baking fish in parchment paper produces a succulent texture and tons of flavor. I love how Mediterranean herbs in this recipe combine with tangy red peppers, sundried tomatoes, and green olives. Guests are sure to swoon at this impressive dinner, even though it's surprisingly easy and quick to make. Serve with my Golden Cauliflower Caesar Salad (page 121) for the perfect meal.

1. Preheat the oven to 400°F.

2. In a small bowl, combine the bell pepper, tomatoes, olives, parsley, avocado oil, capers, garlic, lemon zest, oregano, onion powder, chili flakes (if using), and black pepper.

3. Lay one square of parchment on the countertop and place one fish fillet on it diagonally. Spread one-fourth of the herbed olive mixture on the top of the fillet, then add 2 or 3 lemon slices. Bring the opposite corners of the parchment together and roll them until you reach the fish, then twist the ends and tuck them under the fish. Repeat to wrap the 3 remaining fillets.

4. Place all 4 packets on a baking sheet and bake for 15 minutes. Unwrap and season with sea salt to taste.

Moroccan Fish Balls in Pepper Sauce

Serves: 4

Prep Time: 30 minutes, plus 20 minutes chilling

Cook Time: 1 hour and 10 minutes

Fish Balls

1 pound black cod

Juice of 1 lemon

2 cloves garlic, peeled

½ small yellow onion, coarsely chopped

2 tablespoons tightly packed fresh parsley leaves

2 tablespoons tightly packed fresh cilantro leaves

1 tablespoon tightly packed fresh mint leaves

1 large pasture-raised egg, beaten

¼ cup ground flaxseed

Grated zest of ½ lemon

1 tablespoon avocado oil

1 teaspoon ground cumin

½ teaspoon sea salt

¼ teaspoon ground white pepper

Pepper Sauce

1 tablespoon avocado oil

1 red bell pepper, stemmed, seeded, and sliced

½ jalapeño, seeded and minced (optional)

These delicious cod balls are made with a unique combination of herbs and spices that create powerful flavors and come with a variety of health benefits. For example, parsley has anticancer and anti-diabetic properties, cilantro is detoxifying, and mint is excellent for digestion. This is a great recipe for people who aren't major seafood lovers as the fish is somewhat disguised in the balls and elevated by the other ingredients.

1. For the fish balls: Rinse the cod, place in a bowl, and squeeze the lemon over the top. Freeze for about 20 minutes so it's firm for chopping. Meanwhile, blend the garlic, onion, parsley, cilantro, and mint in a food processor until finely chopped. Remove and set aside in a mixing bowl.

2. Remove the cod from the freezer, rinse again, and dry with paper towels. In a food processor, pulse the fish until it reaches a ground beef–like texture, making sure it doesn't turn into a paste.

3. Combine the cod with the herb mixture, egg, flaxseed, lemon zest, avocado oil, cumin, salt, and white pepper. Mix well, cover, and set aside in the refrigerator.

4. For the pepper sauce: Heat a shallow Dutch oven or a large saucepan over medium heat. Add the avocado oil, bell pepper, and jalapeño (if using) and cook, stirring, until soft, about 5 minutes. Add the cherry tomatoes, reduce the heat to low, and cook for 5 minutes.

5. Add the minced garlic and cook for 8 minutes, continuing to stir. Add the cumin, paprika, hot paprika, turmeric, coriander, cinnamon, and tomato paste and continue to cook and stir for 2 minutes.

6. Add the water, salt, and white pepper and bring to a boil. Reduce the heat, cover, and simmer for 30 minutes.

7. While the sauce is simmering, remove the fish mixture from the refrigerator. Use hands to form 2-tablespoon portions into balls. Once the sauce has simmered for 30 minutes, add all fish balls to the sauce. Cover again, and cook for 35 minutes, stirring occasionally, until the fish balls are hot and cooked through.

1 pint cherry tomatoes
(a variety of colors is best),
halved

4 cloves garlic, minced

1½ teaspoons ground cumin

1½ teaspoons paprika

1 teaspoon hot paprika

½ teaspoon ground turmeric

¼ teaspoon ground coriander

¼ teaspoon ground cinnamon

1 tablespoon tomato paste

1½ cups hot filtered water

½ teaspoon sea salt

½ teaspoon ground white
pepper

Zucchini Noodles

2 medium zucchini

1 tablespoon avocado oil

2 cloves garlic, minced

Pinch of sea salt

Pinch of freshly ground
black pepper

Garnish

¼ cup loosely packed fresh
cilantro, chopped

Juice of ½ lemon

8. For the noodles: While the fish balls cook, spiralize the zucchini to create noodles. Heat the avocado oil in a large pan over medium-high heat until shimmering. Add the minced garlic and sauté for 30 seconds. Add the zucchini noodles, season with the salt and pepper, and cook for 4 minutes, stirring often, until warm but al dente. Remove from the heat and drain off any water that may have seeped into the pan.

9. Divide the noodles among four plates and top with fish balls, scooping sauce onto each. Top with cilantro and a squeeze of lemon juice.

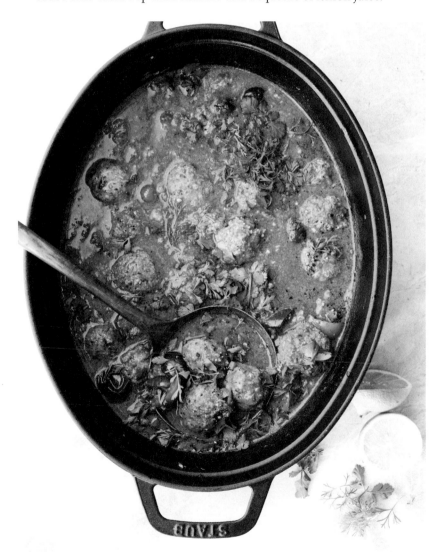

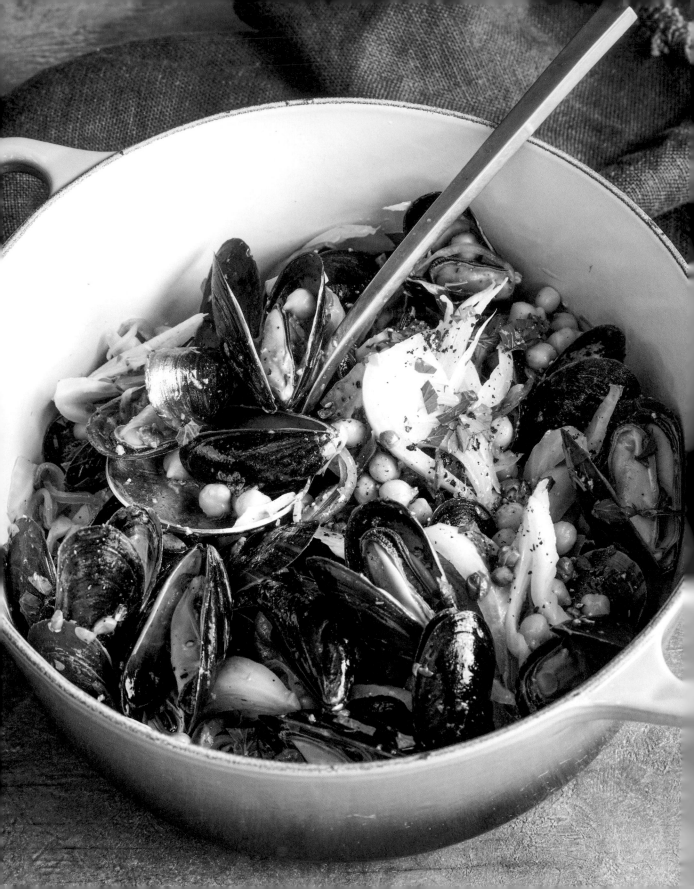

Mussels and Fennel in White Wine

Serves: 4

Prep Time: 15 minutes,
plus 15 minutes soaking

Cook Time: 20 minutes

¼ cup sea salt, plus more
for seasoning

3 cups cold water

4 dozen cleaned debearded
mussels (look for tightly closed
shells with no cracks)

1½ tablespoons avocado oil

1 large red onion, thinly sliced
(about 1½ cups)

¾ cup thinly sliced fennel

2 teaspoons pressed garlic

Grated zest of 1 lemon

2½ tablespoons capers,
rinsed and minced

¾ cup canned chickpeas,
drained and rinsed

1¼ cups loosely packed fresh
parsley leaves, finely chopped

1½ tablespoons lemon juice

Freshly cracked black pepper

1¼ cups Chardonnay

1½ tablespoons ghee or
coconut oil

Mussels are a rich source of a variety of minerals—like selenium, which is essential for optimal thyroid health and a strong immune system. Their slightly briny flavor is balanced perfectly by white wine, fennel, and parsley in a tasty broth. Chickpeas add extra protein and fiber. For a complete meal and an extra pop of color, serve with my Roasted Beet and Citrus Salad (page 127).

1. In a large bowl or pot, mix ¼ cup salt with the cold water. Add the mussels and let soak for 15 minutes in the fridge. Drain.

2. Heat the avocado oil in a large pot over medium heat until shimmering. Add the onion and fennel and sauté for 7 minutes, until the onion is translucent. Add the garlic, lemon zest, capers, and ¼ teaspoon salt. Stir well for 1 minute. Add the chickpeas and cook for 4 minutes, stirring occasionally.

3. Add the drained mussels, parsley, lemon juice, and cracked pepper. Mix thoroughly, then add the wine and ghee. Turn the heat to medium-high, cover the pot, and cook for 5 minutes. Check to see if most of the mussels have opened. If they haven't, cover and continue to cook, checking every minute, for up to 7 minutes total. Remove the pan from the heat and discard any mussels that haven't opened. Serve right away.

Slow-Roasted Salmon with Mustard Glaze

CONTRIBUTED BY LEIZE PERLMUTTER AND DAVID PERLMUTTER, MD

Serves: 4

Prep Time: 15 minutes
Cook Time: 20 minutes

¼ cup plus 2 tablespoons
unsalted grass-fed butter,
at room temperature (plus
more for greasing the pan)

¼ cup raw almonds, finely
ground

2 tablespoons tightly packed
chopped fresh flat-leaf parsley

2 teaspoons Dijon mustard

1 teaspoon mustard seeds

1 teaspoon grated lemon zest

4 (5-ounce) skinless wild-
caught salmon fillets

Sea salt and freshly ground
black pepper

This delectable salmon dish comes from my friends Leize Perlmutter and Dr. David Perlmutter, pioneers in the realm of nutrition and brain health. Adapted from *The Grain Brain Cookbook*, it's a nourishing dish that promotes optimal brain function from the omega-3 fatty acids found in grass-fed butter and wild-caught salmon. It also provides beneficial phytonutrients from fresh parsley and almonds.

1. Preheat the oven to 275°F. Generously butter a shallow baking dish large enough to hold the fillets without crowding.

2. In a small bowl, combine the butter, almonds, parsley, mustard, mustard seeds, and lemon zest and use a rubber spatula to knead and blend thoroughly. Spread an equal portion of the butter mixture over the top of each salmon fillet. Season with salt and pepper, then transfer to the roasting pan.

3. Roast the salmon in the oven until the fish is barely cooked through and the top is glazed, about 20 minutes. Remove from the oven and serve.

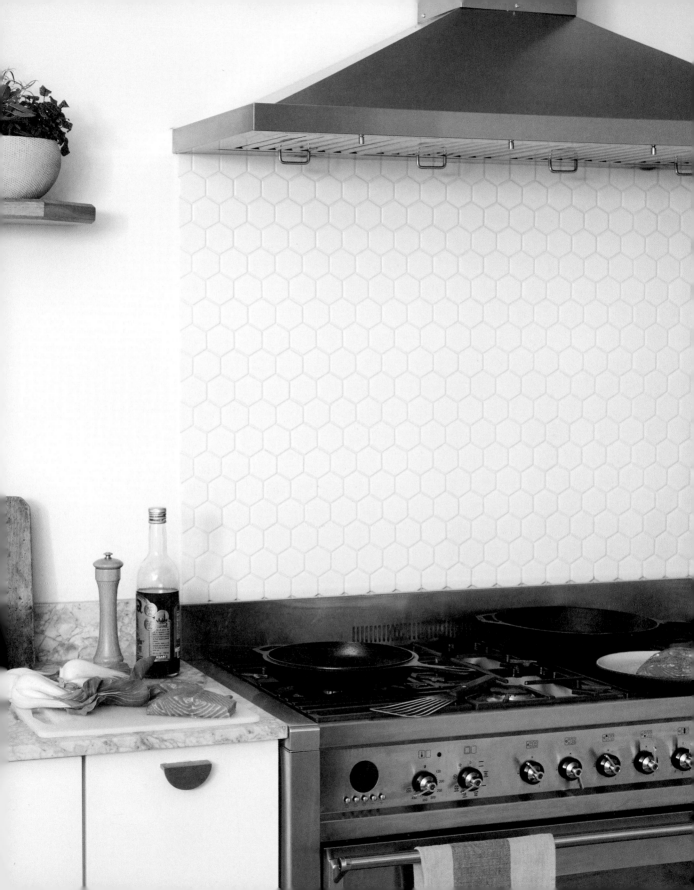

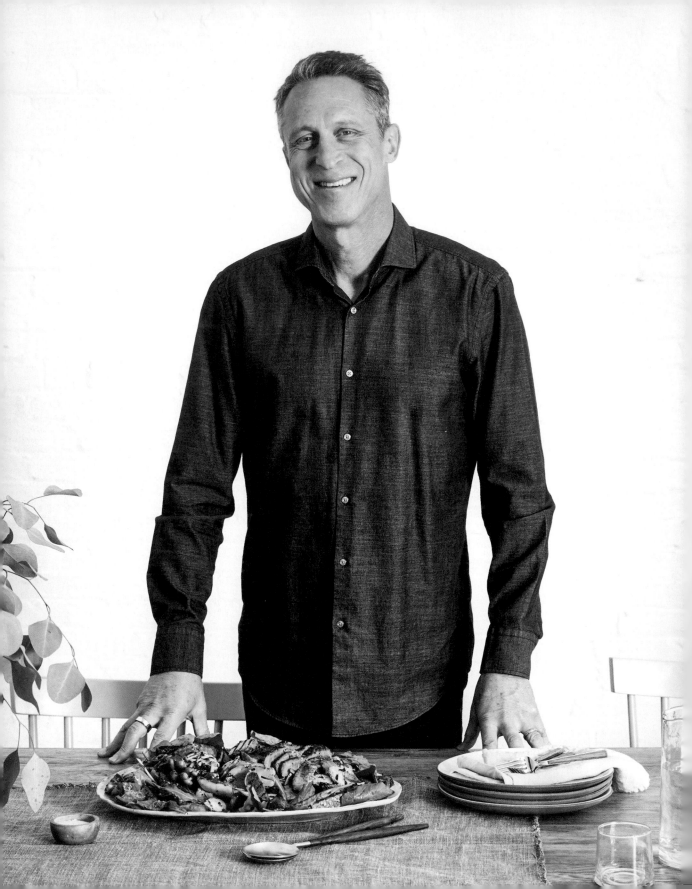

Beef and Lamb

Red meat was villainized for far too long. The key to enjoying it consciously is to buy grass-fed cuts for maximum nutrition and minimal environmental impact. These meat dishes are bursting with a variety of fresh herbs and spices and complemented by plenty of colorful vegetables; you're sure to love them.

Bison Wraps with Poblano-Avocado Sauce

Serves: 4 (3 small wraps per serving)

Prep Time: 35 minutes, plus 1 hour marinating

Cook Time: 30 minutes

Steak and Marinade

¼ cup plus 2 tablespoons avocado oil

¼ cup plus 2 tablespoons lime juice

2 teaspoons minced seeded jalapeño

2 teaspoons sea salt, plus more for seasoning

2 teaspoons garlic powder

1 teaspoon chili powder, plus more for seasoning

1 teaspoon smoked paprika

Pinch of freshly ground black pepper, plus more for seasoning

3 (6-ounce) bison strip steaks

Poblano-Avocado Sauce

½ medium poblano pepper, stemmed and seeded

1 large shallot, peeled

1 tablespoon plus 1 teaspoon avocado oil

3 small tomatillos, papery husks removed, chopped (about ½ cup)

¼ cup chopped avocado

¼ cup plus 1 tablespoon loosely packed fresh cilantro, finely minced

It's easy to make a wrap extra nutritious by swapping out the flour tortillas for collard greens and the cheese for a creamy avocado sauce. Bison is an amazing lean protein source that takes collard wraps to the next level. It's rich in vitamin B$_{12}$ and minerals like zinc, and it is almost always grass-fed, so you can feel confident that you're getting high-quality meat.

1. For the steak and marinade: Mix all the ingredients for the marinade in a shallow dish. Add the steaks and turn to coat. Cover and marinate in the fridge for 1 hour.

2. Preheat the oven to 425°F.

3. For the poblano sauce: Place the poblano pepper and shallot on a baking sheet and drizzle with 1 teaspoon of the avocado oil, coating well. Roast, flipping halfway through, for 20 minutes, until tender and fragrant. Let cool slightly, then peel the skin from the poblano pepper. Put the pepper and shallot in a high-speed blender along with the remaining 1 tablespoon avocado oil, the tomatillos, avocado, cilantro, jalapeño, garlic, lime juice, smoked paprika, onion powder, and salt and blend until smooth.

4. To trim the collard greens of the thick central vein that begins about halfway down the leaf and turns into the stem: Lay each leaf flat on a cutting board and carefully run a paring knife down one side of the thickest part of the central vein (cut with knife moving away from your body). Repeat on the other side of the vein, then cut and discard the stem.

5. Prepare a large bowl of ice water; bring 5 cups of water to a boil in a large pot. One at a time, blanch the collard leaves in the boiling water for 30 seconds, then immediately submerge in the ice bath for 10 seconds. Place on paper towels to dry.

1½ teaspoons minced seeded jalapeño (optional)

½ teaspoon pressed garlic

1 tablespoon plus 1 teaspoon lime juice

¼ teaspoon smoked paprika

¼ teaspoon onion powder

¾ teaspoon sea salt

Collard Wraps and Vegetables

12 leaves collard greens

1 tablespoon avocado oil

1 medium red onion, finely chopped (about 1 cup)

1 teaspoon ground cumin

1½ teaspoons sea salt

1½ cups shredded purple cabbage

½ red bell pepper, stemmed, seeded, and thinly sliced

½ yellow bell pepper, stemmed, seeded, and thinly sliced

½ orange bell pepper, stemmed, seeded, and thinly sliced

2 medium zucchini, quartered lengthwise and sliced into ¼-inch triangles (about 2 cups)

¾ cup loosely packed fresh cilantro, minced

Juice of 1 lime

6. Heat a grill or grill pan to medium-high.

7. For the vegetables: Heat the avocado oil in a large sauté pan over medium-high heat until shimmering. Add the onion, cumin, and salt and sauté for 8 minutes. Add the cabbage and sauté for 2 minutes. Reduce the heat to medium and add the bell peppers. Stir well and sauté for 7 minutes. Add the zucchini, cilantro, and lime juice and stir well. Continue cooking for about 5 minutes, until the zucchini is cooked through but still firm.

8. Remove the steaks from the marinade and sprinkle both sides with additional salt, pepper, and chili powder. Grill until desired doneness, or about 5 minutes per side for medium. Set aside to cool slightly, then cut into thin slices.

9. To serve, place sliced steak, vegetables, and poblano sauce on each collard leaf and wrap like a burrito.

Eggplant Moussaka

This incredible, comforting dish is perfect for feeding a crowd. Tender eggplant and sweet potato slices are layered with a savory meat sauce and creamy béchamel, then baked into one bubbly, beautiful meal. The moussaka is rich in protein, fiber, and antioxidants like beta-carotene, and it makes for excellent leftovers. Store covered in the fridge for up to 3 days; reheat at 400°F for 15 minutes, or until the béchamel is bubbling.

Serves: 6

Prep Time: 25 minutes, plus 15 minutes cooling

Cook Time: 1½ hours

Veggie Layers

3 tablespoons avocado oil, plus more for the pan

1 small Hannah sweet potato

2 medium eggplants, cut lengthwise into ½-inch-thick slices

Meat Sauce

2 tablespoons avocado oil

1 large white onion, minced

1 Fresno chile, seeded and minced

4 large cloves garlic, minced

½ pound ground lamb

½ pound grass-fed ground beef

1 tablespoon smoked paprika

1½ teaspoons ground cumin

1 teaspoon ground cinnamon

1 tablespoon pink Himalayan salt or sea salt

1 tablespoon freshly ground black pepper

6 tablespoons tomato paste

1 tomato, seeded and chopped

2 tablespoons tightly packed chopped fresh mint

2 tablespoons tightly packed chopped fresh oregano

Coconut Béchamel

2 tablespoons ghee

1. Preheat the oven to 425°F. Line a large baking sheet with parchment paper and grease a casserole dish with avocado oil.

2. For the veggies: Cut the sweet potato into ¼-inch-thick rounds and set aside. Place the eggplant slices and 3 tablespoons avocado oil in a large, shallow bowl and mix until the eggplant is saturated. Transfer to the lined baking sheet, arrange in a single layer, and roast until tender and browned, 35 to 45 minutes. Remove and reduce the oven temperature to 400°F.

3. For the meat sauce: Heat the avocado oil in a large pot over medium-high heat until shimmering. Add the onion and sauté until tender, 5 to 8 minutes. Add the chile and garlic and sauté for 5 minutes. Add the lamb, beef, smoked paprika, cumin, cinnamon, salt, and pepper and cook until the meat is fully cooked, about 7 minutes. Add the tomato paste and chopped tomato and cook until all the liquid has evaporated, about 7 minutes. Add the mint and oregano, stir for 2 minutes, then turn off heat.

4. For the béchamel: In a saucepan, melt the ghee over medium heat until hot, then add the almond flour; whisk constantly until fully combined. Whisk in the coconut milk and bring to a boil. Add the nutmeg and black pepper and cook, stirring, for about 5 minutes, until the mixture thickens. Remove from the heat and quickly stir in the egg yolks, one by one.

1 cup almond flour

1 (15-ounce) can full-fat unsweetened coconut milk

1½ teaspoons ground nutmeg

1½ teaspoons freshly ground black pepper

2 large pasture-raised egg yolks

5. To assemble the moussaka, cover the bottom of the casserole dish with all of the raw sweet potato rounds. Top with half of the sliced roasted eggplant, then half of the meat sauce, then half of the béchamel. Make three more layers with the eggplant, meat sauce, and then the béchamel on top.

6. Cover and bake for 20 minutes. Uncover and bake for an additional 20 to 25 minutes, until the top layer of béchamel is lightly browned. Let cool for 15 minutes before cutting.

Sweet Potato UnBuns

1½ teaspoons avocado oil

4 cups grated peeled sweet potatoes (about 1 pound)

2 cups grated zucchini (3 to 4 medium)

⅓ cup thinly sliced green onions

1½ teaspoons ground ginger

½ teaspoon sea salt

3 large pasture-raised eggs

Sliders

1 pound grass-fed ground beef

1 tablespoon extra virgin olive oil

1 tablespoon tightly packed minced fresh rosemary

1 tablespoon tightly packed minced fresh thyme

1 tablespoon tightly packed minced fresh sage

1 tablespoon tightly packed minced fresh oregano

1 tablespoon tightly packed minced fresh parsley

1 teaspoon sea salt, plus more for seasoning

1 tablespoon avocado oil

Garnish

5 red radishes, thinly sliced

3 green onions, cut into thin ribbons

3 avocados, pitted, peeled, and thinly sliced

Grass-Fed Sliders on Sweet Potato UnBuns

CONTRIBUTED BY DAVE ASPREY

Shredded sweet potatoes create the most amazing grain-less bun for these savory, juicy burgers, which are a Team Hyman favorite. My good friend Dave Asprey, founder of Bulletproof 360, Inc., was kind enough to share these mouthwatering sliders from his very own Bulletproof Café. I know you'll love them as much as we do.

1. For the unbuns: Preheat the oven to 350°F; line two large baking sheets with parchment paper, then grease them with the avocado oil.

2. In a colander over the sink, squeeze the grated sweet potato and zucchini tightly to release any extra water. This can be done by hand or by using a piece of cheesecloth. Transfer to a large bowl, add the green onions, ginger, and salt, and toss. Add the eggs and mix well with hands. Shape the mixture into 20 small patties, using about 3 tablespoons for each, and place, evenly spaced, on the baking sheets.

3. Bake for 20 minutes. Rotate the pans between the top and bottom oven racks and bake for another 20 to 25 minutes, until the buns are firm and golden brown around the edges. Let cool completely before removing from the pan.

4. While the buns are baking, make the sliders: Heat a grill or grill pan to medium heat.

5. Place the ground beef in a large bowl and add the olive oil, rosemary, thyme, sage, oregano, parsley, and salt. Using your fingers like a pitchfork, mix gently. Be careful not to overmix. Shape the mixture into 10 small patties, using about 3 tablespoons meat per patty.

6. Brush the grill with the avocado oil to prevent sliders from sticking, then place the patties on the grill and cook for 6 minutes. Flip and cook for another 4 to 6 minutes for medium, or longer to your desired temperature.

7. Remove sliders from the grill and sprinkle with additional sea salt. Serve each between two sweet potato buns, topped with sliced radish and green onion ribbons, with avocado on the side.

Serves: 4

Prep Time: 15 minutes, plus 30 marinating

Cook Time: 30 minutes

Lamb and Marinade

3 tablespoons avocado oil

2 tablespoons red wine vinegar

2 tablespoons coconut aminos

1 tablespoon pressed garlic

1½ teaspoons ground cumin

¼ teaspoon smoked paprika

½ teaspoon sea salt

1¼ pounds grass-fed lamb shoulder, cut into 1½-inch cubes

Carrots

8 medium carrots

2 tablespoons minced green onion, plus more for garnish

2 tablespoons avocado oil

1 tablespoon lemon juice

½ teaspoon onion powder

¼ teaspoon smoked paprika

½ teaspoon sea salt

Tahini Sauce

½ cup tahini

¼ cup filtered water

2 tablespoons lemon juice

2 tablespoons coconut aminos

2 teaspoons ground cumin

2 teaspoons pressed garlic

½ teaspoon sea salt

Lamb Skewers with Roasted Carrots

Lamb is a delicious way to switch up your animal proteins, and grass-fed lamb is also a great source of immune-boosting zinc. These tender skewers pair nicely with savory roasted carrots and a rich tahini sauce for a colorful plate. The cumin provides polyphenols and promotes good digestion.

1. Preheat the oven to 375°F; line a baking sheet with parchment paper. If grilling the lamb, soak 8 bamboo skewers in water for 30 minutes.

2. For the lamb and marinade: Mix the marinade ingredients in a bowl. Add the lamb, toss to coat, cover, and marinate in the fridge for 30 minutes.

3. For the carrots: Wash the carrots well and cut off the tops. Cut crosswise into 4 pieces, then cut into matchsticks. In a bowl, toss the carrots with the green onion, avocado oil, lemon juice, onion powder, smoked paprika, and salt. Arrange on the lined baking sheet and roast for 30 minutes, until fork tender.

4. For the sauce: Combine the tahini, water, lemon juice, coconut aminos, cumin, garlic, and salt in a medium bowl and whisk together well.

5. While the carrots are cooking, cook the lamb: If using a grill or grill pan, heat to medium. Thread the lamb cubes onto the soaked skewers. Grill the lamb for 4 minutes, then turn and grill another 4 minutes for medium. If using the oven, place the lamb cubes on a wire rack and place the rack in a parchment-lined baking sheet. Roast with the carrots in the 375°F oven for 5 minutes, then flip the cubes and roast another 5 minutes for medium, or until desired doneness.

6. To serve, spread the tahini sauce on a large platter and arrange the carrots and lamb on top. Garnish with additional green onions.

Middle Eastern Lamb Liver with Parsley Salad

CONTRIBUTED BY TERRY WAHLS, MD

Serves: 4

Prep Time: 10 minutes
Cook Time: 4 minutes

1 medium red onion,
quartered and sliced

1 bunch fresh parsley, minced

1 to 2 tablespoons ground
sumac (or pomegranate seeds)

3 tablespoons extra virgin
olive oil

1 tablespoon balsamic vinegar

1 tablespoon ghee or
extra virgin olive oil

1 tablespoon apple cider
vinegar

½ to 1 teaspoon ground cumin

1 pound grass-fed lamb liver,
thinly sliced

Sea salt and freshly ground
black pepper

Liver is ultra-rich in a variety of nutrients, like the fat-soluble vitamins A, D, and K as well as vitamin B$_{12}$ and minerals like zinc and copper. My friend Dr. Terry Wahls, author of *The Wahls Protocol Cooking for Life*, was able to reverse the progression of her multiple sclerosis using food as medicine. She shared this recipe as it's one of her family's favorites and takes no time at all to make.

1. In a medium bowl, toss the onion and parsley together. Add the sumac, olive oil, and balsamic vinegar and mix well.

2. Melt the ghee in a large skillet over low heat. Add the cider vinegar, increase the heat to medium, and cook until steaming. Stir in the cumin. Add the liver, cover, and cook for 1 to 2 minutes. Flip the liver, cover, and cook 1 to 2 minutes longer, until no longer pink. Remove from the heat and allow to sit, covered, for 5 minutes. (The goal is to have the liver rare or medium-rare. If the liver is well-done it will be tough.)

3. Season with salt and pepper to taste and serve with the parsley salad.

Shepherd's Pie with Sweet Potato Topping

CONTRIBUTED BY DREW RAMSEY, MD

Serves: 6

Prep Time: 25 minutes
Cook Time: 40 minutes

3 pounds sweet potatoes (about 3 large potatoes), peeled and quartered

1 tablespoon extra virgin olive oil

1 large onion, chopped (about 1½ cups)

5 ounces mushrooms (such as cremini, button, or shiitake), chopped

1 pound grass-fed ground beef

½ cup cooked lentils

1 tablespoon gluten-free Worcestershire sauce

¼ teaspoon freshly ground black pepper, or other seasoning of choice

⅔ cup full-fat unsweetened coconut milk

1 teaspoon garlic powder

1 teaspoon baking powder

This comforting recipe was shared by my friend Dr. Drew Ramsey, a nutritional psychiatrist and author. His nutrient-dense version of shepherd's pie combines a savory protein-rich base of lentils, mushrooms, and grass-fed beef with a topping of perfect golden puréed sweet potatoes. This is a colorful and satisfying meal to serve a crowd.

1. Preheat the oven to 400°F.

2. Put the potatoes in a medium pot, cover with water by at least 1 inch, and bring to a boil. Reduce the heat and simmer until tender, 12 to 15 minutes.

3. While the potatoes are cooking, warm the olive oil in a large skillet over medium heat. When shimmering, add the onion and mushrooms and cook until tender, 5 to 6 minutes. Push the vegetables to the side of the pan and add the beef. Brown for 2 to 3 minutes without stirring. Continue to cook, breaking up the meat, for about 2 minutes longer. Stir in the lentils, Worcestershire sauce, and pepper. Transfer the beef and vegetable mixture to a 7x11-inch baking dish.

4. Once the potatoes are fork-tender, drain and transfer to a food processor. Add the coconut milk and garlic powder and process until smooth. Sprinkle the baking powder over the mixture and process again to incorporate. Using a spatula, evenly spread the potato mixture over the meat mixture in the baking dish.

5. Bake for 35 to 40 minutes, until the pie is bubbling hot and the top is golden. Let cool 5 minutes before serving.

Serves: 4

Prep Time: 15 minutes, plus 1 hour marinating

Cook Time: 15 to 20 minutes

Steaks and Marinade

¼ cup plus 3 tablespoons avocado oil

2 tablespoons balsamic vinegar

1 tablespoon ginger juice (pressed from 2 tablespoons grated fresh ginger)

1 teaspoon garlic powder

¼ teaspoon chili flakes

1 teaspoon sea salt

4 (6-ounce) grass-fed rib eye steaks

1 tablespoon fresh cracked pepper

Oyster Mushrooms

1 pound oyster mushrooms

2 tablespoons ghee

1 teaspoon sea salt, plus more for seasoning

2 teaspoons freshly ground black pepper

1 cup thinly sliced green onions (about 2 bunches)

2 large cloves garlic, minced

15 leaves fresh tarragon

½ tablespoon tightly packed fresh thyme leaves

1 tablespoon sherry vinegar

1 pinch Maldon salt

Peppered Steaks with Roasted Oyster Mushrooms

The combination of juicy steak and gorgeous roasted oyster mushrooms is ultra-comforting and satisfying. Grass-fed steak is rich in iron, B-vitamins, zinc, and selenium, while oyster mushrooms contain a powerful antioxidant called ergothioneine, which can ease systemic inflammation and reduce the risk of cardiovascular disease.

1. Make the marinade for the steak by combining ¼ cup plus 2 tablespoons of the avocado oil, the balsamic vinegar, ginger juice, garlic powder, chili flakes, and ½ teaspoon of the salt in a large wide bowl. Add the steak and turn to coat well. Cover and marinate in the fridge for 1 hour.

2. Preheat the oven to 375°F.

3. Remove the steak from the marinade and pat dry with paper towels. Rub ½ tablespoon of the remaining avocado oil over the steaks and season with the remaining ½ teaspoon sea salt. Press the fresh cracked pepper into both sides of the steaks.

4. Heat the remaining ½ tablespoon avocado oil in a large cast-iron pan over high heat. Sear each side of the steaks for 2 minutes and the edges for 30 seconds. Transfer the pan to the oven and roast for 7 minutes for medium doneness. Cook longer if desired. Loosely tent the pan with foil and let the steaks rest. Increase the oven temperature to 400°F.

5. For the mushrooms: Cut away the woody base of the main mushroom stem and use your hands to separate the individual mushrooms into pieces.

6. Heat the ghee in a large cast-iron skillet over medium-high heat. Add the mushrooms and season with the salt and pepper. Cook without stirring until browned, about 4 minutes. Transfer the skillet to the 400°F oven and roast the mushrooms for 5 minutes. Add the green

onions and garlic, toss the mushrooms, and roast for another 6 to 8 minutes, until golden and tender. Add the tarragon, thyme, and sherry vinegar and toss. Add a pinch of Maldon salt on top.

7. Cut the steaks into thin strips and serve with a heap of roasted mushrooms. Season with more salt and pepper to taste.

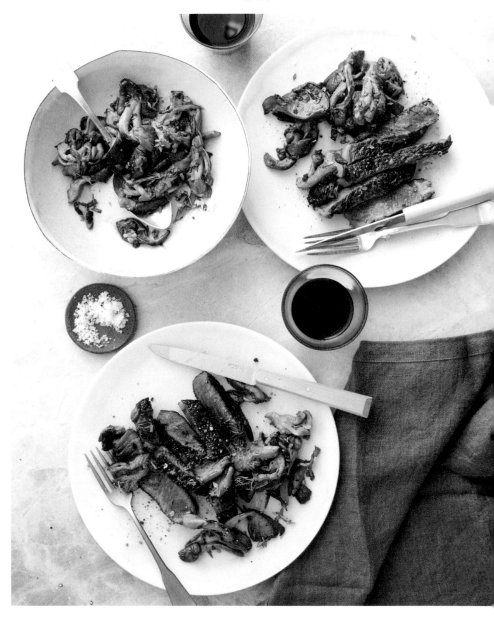

Slow-Cooked Lamb with Minty Millet

Serves: 6

Prep Time: 20 minutes
Cook Time: 3½ hours (or 6 hours in the slow cooker)

Lamb

2 pounds grass-fed bone-in lamb shoulder

1½ teaspoons sea salt

½ teaspoon freshly ground black pepper

1 tablespoon avocado oil

2 teaspoons ground cumin

1 teaspoon ground coriander

½ teaspoon ground ginger

½ teaspoon ground turmeric

½ teaspoon onion powder

¼ teaspoon cayenne

¼ teaspoon ground cinnamon

1 large white onion, chopped (about 2 cups)

1 (13.5-ounce) can diced tomatoes

1 tablespoon plus 1 teaspoon pressed garlic

1 tablespoon lemon juice

2 medium zucchini, cut into ¼-inch half-moons (about 4 cups)

This lamb will fall right off the bone and melt deliciously in your mouth, thanks to the added moisture and intense flavor from slow cooking. Cumin, coriander, and cinnamon contribute exotic and warming spice, while millet and cauliflower with a dose of mint add contrasting flavor and texture to soak up the stewed veggies. Lamb is rich in protein, along with B$_{12}$ and iron, so it's especially helpful for maintaining healthy blood cells.

1. For the lamb: Preheat the oven to 300°F. Season the lamb with salt and pepper. Heat the avocado oil in a large cast-iron skillet over medium heat until shimmering. Lightly sear each side of the lamb, about 3 minutes per side, until browned.

2. Transfer the lamb to a Dutch oven. Add all the spices, along with the onion, tomatoes, garlic, and lemon juice. Stir well, cover, and bake in the oven for 3 hours. Add the zucchini and cook for another 30 minutes. The meat should be falling off the bone. (Alternatively, you can cook the lamb, spices, onions, tomatoes, garlic, and lemon juice in a slow cooker on low for 5 hours. Then add the zucchini and cook for another 30 to 60 minutes.)

3. Meanwhile, toast the nuts for the millet: Toast the pine nuts in a medium sauté pan over medium-high heat, continuously stirring and shaking, until fragrant and golden, about 3 minutes. Remove from the heat and set aside.

4. When the lamb has about 35 minutes left, combine the millet and water in a large pot and bring it to a boil over medium-high heat. Cover, reduce the heat to as low as possible, and simmer for 20 minutes, until the water is absorbed.

Millet

¾ cup pine nuts

¾ cup millet

1½ cups filtered water

1½ cups riced cauliflower

¾ cup finely chopped
fresh mint

3 teaspoons lemon zest

1 tablespoon plus 1 teaspoon
lemon juice

2 teaspoons avocado oil

1 teaspoon sea salt

5. In a bowl, combine ½ cup of the pine nuts, the cauliflower, ½ cup of the mint, 1 teaspoon of the lemon zest, the lemon juice, avocado oil, and salt. Immediately stir the cauliflower mixture into the millet in the pot and remove the pot from the heat. Set aside, covered, so the warm millet can steam the cauliflower.

6. To serve, use two forks to pull the lamb off the bone. Divide the millet mixture among six bowls and top evenly with shredded lamb and stewed vegetables. Use the remaining ¼ cup mint, ¼ cup pine nuts, and 2 teaspoons lemon zest to garnish bowls evenly.

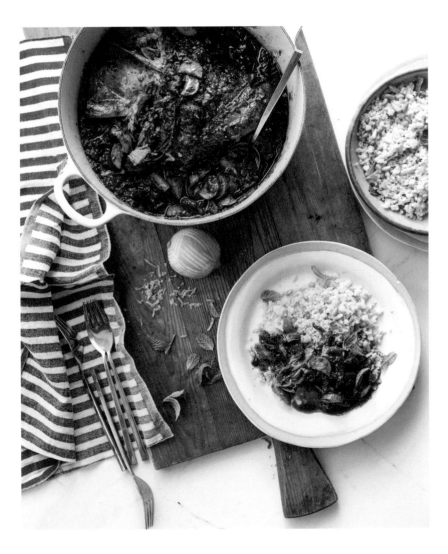

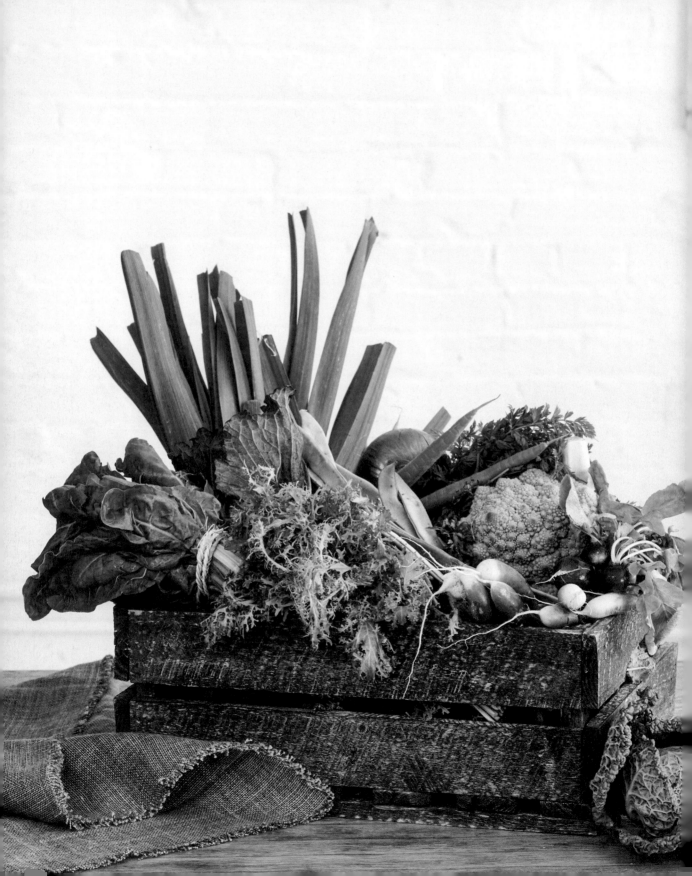

Veggies

One of the best things you can do for your health is eat the rainbow every day. The colorful vegetables that make up these entrées provide a variety of beneficial phytonutrients and antioxidants, plus plant-based protein and plenty of healthy fats. These beautiful meals look as good as they make you feel.

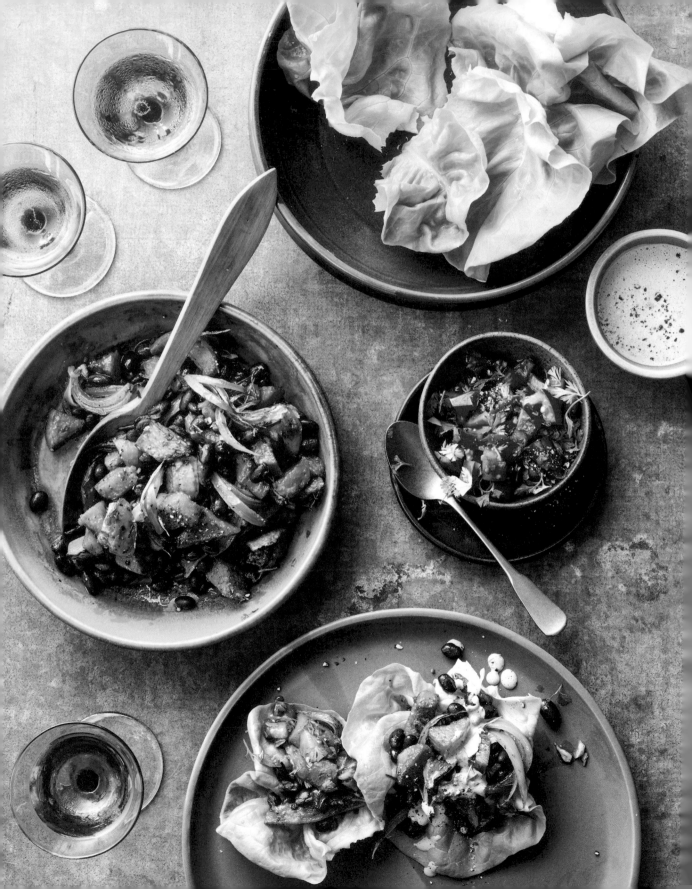

Serves: 4

Prep Time: 15 minutes
Cook Time: 30 minutes

Taco Filling

1 (1-pound) butternut squash,
peeled, seeded, and cut into
large cubes

1 large yellow onion, cut into
¼-inch slices

2 tablespoons avocado oil

1 teaspoon dried oregano

¼ teaspoon chipotle powder

1 teaspoon sea salt

1 cup canned black beans,
rinsed and drained

Hemp Seed Cream

¼ cup hemp seeds

1 tablespoon minced fresh mint

1 teaspoon pressed garlic

2 tablespoons lime juice

2 tablespoons filtered water

1 tablespoon extra virgin
olive oil

¼ teaspoon smoked paprika

½ teaspoon sea salt

Salsa

1 large tomato, seeded and
diced

½ cup loosely packed fresh
cilantro leaves, roughly
chopped

Grated zest and juice of 1 lime

½ teaspoon sea salt

To Serve

1 large head butter lettuce,
leaves removed from the core

Butternut Taco Wraps with Hemp Seed Cream

Sweet-and-savory, vegan, grain-free: These tacos are a tasty alternative to traditional ones laden with dairy and wheat. Tender butter lettuce makes a great alternative to taco shells, while butternut squash and black beans combine for a delicious, antioxidant-rich filling. Hemp seeds blend into a delightfully smooth sauce to add a creamy dollop of texture along with a nice dose of omega-3 fatty acids.

1. Preheat the oven to 425°F.

2. For the filling: Combine the squash, onion, avocado oil, oregano, chipotle powder, and salt. Toss well and spread out on a baking sheet. Roast for 20 to 25 minutes, until the squash is tender.

3. Warm the beans in a small skillet over medium heat. Add to the squash mixture and keep warm.

4. For the hemp cream: Combine the hemp seeds, mint, garlic, lime juice, water, olive oil, smoked paprika, and salt in a small food processor and blend until smooth.

5. For the salsa: Combine the tomato, cilantro, lime zest and juice, and salt in a small bowl and stir well.

6. To serve, fill each lettuce leaf with the squash filling. Top with a dollop of cream and salsa.

Creamy Truffle Spaghetti Squash with Tempeh

Serves: 4

Prep Time: 15 minutes, plus 30 minutes marinating

Cook Time: 50 minutes

Tempeh and Marinade

¼ cup gluten-free tamari

1 tablespoon avocado oil

1 tablespoon balsamic vinegar

1 teaspoon garlic powder

1 teaspoon onion powder

1 teaspoon dried oregano

½ teaspoon smoked paprika

2 (8-ounce) packages gluten-free tempeh, cut into cubes

Spaghetti Squash

2 small or 1 large spaghetti squash (about 6 cups cooked)

1 tablespoon plus 1 teaspoon avocado oil

¼ teaspoon sea salt

¼ teaspoon freshly ground black pepper

Spaghetti squash is an amazing replacement for traditional pasta. Rich in fiber, vitamin C, and vitamin B₆, it's a much healthier option than highly refined, wheat-based noodles. Toasted pine nuts blend into a nutty, creamy sauce that is taken to the next level with a drizzle of robust black truffle oil.

1. To marinate the tempeh: Mix the tamari, avocado oil, vinegar, garlic powder, onion powder, oregano, and smoked paprika in a medium bowl. Add the tempeh pieces and turn to coat with the marinade; let sit for 30 minutes at room temperature.

2. For the squash: Preheat the oven to 375°F; line a baking sheet with parchment paper.

3. Cut the squash in half and remove the seeds. Rub the avocado oil on the cut sides of the halves. Sprinkle the salt and pepper evenly over the oiled areas. Place facedown on the lined baking sheet. Roast the squash until the skin can be pierced through with a fork and the flesh is tender, 25 to 40 minutes, depending on the size of your squash (be sure to check it at 25 minutes). Let cool before touching the flesh.

4. While the squash cooks, make the pine nut cream: Heat a medium sauté pan over medium-high heat. Add the pine nuts and toast, stirring frequently, until the seeds are fragrant and toasted, about 3 minutes.

5. In a small food processor, combine the toasted pine nuts, water, truffle oil, green onions, parsley, olive oil, lemon zest, garlic, salt, and pepper and blend until smooth.

Pine Nut Cream

¾ cup pine nuts

½ cup filtered water

¼ cup black truffle oil, plus
4 teaspoons for serving

¼ cup chopped green onions

¼ cup loosely packed fresh
parsley, plus more for garnish

¼ cup extra virgin olive oil

Grated zest of 4 lemons
(about 2 tablespoons)

2 teaspoons pressed garlic

1 teaspoon sea salt

1 teaspoon freshly ground
black pepper

To Finish

2 tablespoons avocado oil

⅓ cup finely chopped shallots

6. To finish the tempeh: Heat 1 tablespoon of the avocado oil in a large pan over medium-low heat until shimmering. Add the shallots and sauté for 6 minutes. Add the remaining 1 tablespoon avocado oil and crumble the cubes of tempeh into the pan. Turn the heat up to medium and sauté the tempeh for 5 minutes. Turn the heat off and add the pine nut cream, stirring well.

7. To serve, scrape the squash strands from the skin and divide among four plates. Drizzle each serving with 1 teaspoon black truffle oil. Top with the tempeh mixture and garnish with additional parsley.

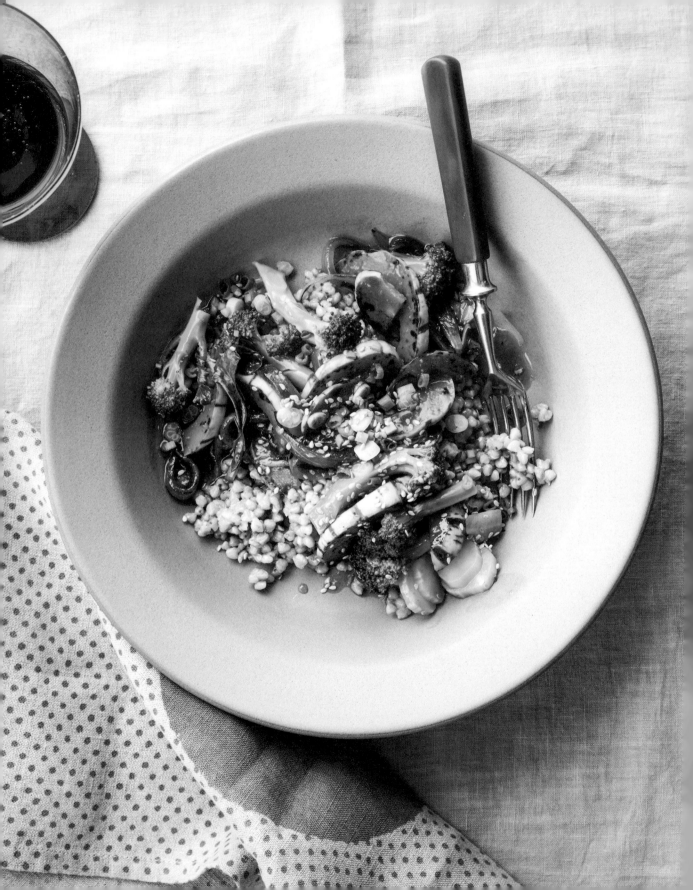

Serves: 4

Prep Time: 10 minutes
Cook Time: 20 minutes

½ cup raw buckwheat groats

1 small head cauliflower, cored and roughly chopped

2 cups filtered water

1 tablespoon coconut oil

2 tablespoons sesame oil

1 small yellow onion, sliced ¼-inch thick

1 small delicata squash, halved, seeded, and cut into ¼-inch half-moons

1 (1-inch) piece fresh ginger, peeled and minced

1 large clove garlic, minced

1 large broccoli head, stems peeled and cut into ¼-inch rounds, florets cut into bite-size pieces

2 cups vegetable broth

2 tablespoons gluten-free tamari

2 tablespoons sesame seeds

¼ cup loosely packed fresh cilantro leaves

Delicata Buckwheat Bowls

Delicata is one of my favorite varieties of squash due to its subtly sweet taste and tender texture—and I love that there is no need to peel it! It's also a good source of beta-carotene and vitamin C. Cook the squash with crunchy broccoli and spoon over hearty buckwheat for a nourishing one-bowl meal that is sure to fill you up, plus it makes for great leftovers. Store any extra in a glass container in the fridge for 2 to 3 days.

1. Rinse the buckwheat under cold water until the water runs clear. Combine the buckwheat in a saucepan with the chopped cauliflower and water, then add the coconut oil and bring to a boil over medium-high heat. Cover, reduce the heat to a simmer, and cook until the water is almost fully absorbed, about 10 minutes. Set aside and let stand for 5 minutes before removing the lid.

2. While the buckwheat cooks, heat a 10-inch skillet over medium-high heat. Add the sesame oil; once shimmering, add the onion, and stir and cook for 1 minute. Add the squash and sauté for 3 minutes.

3. Add the ginger and garlic, stir to combine, and cook until fragrant, about 3 minutes. Add the broccoli, broth, and tamari, cover, and cook for 5 minutes, until the broccoli is tender.

4. To serve, divide the buckwheat/cauliflower mixture among four bowls, then spoon the squash/broccoli mixture on top. Garnish with sesame seeds and cilantro and serve.

Forbidden Rice No-Fry Stir-Fry

Serves: 4

Prep Time: 15 minutes
Cook Time: 40 minutes

½ cup black wild rice (also called Forbidden Rice), rinsed

1½ cups filtered water

¼ cup slivered raw almonds

2 tablespoons avocado oil

1 small yellow onion, thinly sliced

1 large head broccoli, stems peeled and sliced paper thin, florets cut into bite-size pieces

1 small carrot, cut into paper-thin rounds

8 white mushrooms, thinly sliced

1 small red bell pepper, stemmed, seeded, and thinly sliced

1 small yellow bell pepper, stemmed, seeded, and thinly sliced

1 small head bok choy, thinly sliced

Stir-fries are a staple of a healthy, home-cooked diet since they allow you to incorporate a variety of vegetables into a nourishing dinner that is quick and easy. This one uses edamame as a plant-based protein; just be sure to choose organic soy to avoid GMOs. All the amazing flavors in this recipe shine against an antioxidant-rich black rice base.

1. Combine the rice and water in a small pot and bring to a boil over medium-high heat. Reduce the heat, cover, and simmer for 25 to 30 minutes, until the rice is tender. Spread on a large plate to cool.

2. Heat a small sauté pan over medium-high heat. Add the slivered almonds and stir frequently until fragrant and toasted, about 5 minutes. Remove from heat and set aside.

3. For the veggies, heat the avocado oil over medium heat in a large sauté pan or wok until shimmering. Add the onion, broccoli stem and florets, and carrots and stir-fry for 5 minutes. Add the mushrooms, bell peppers, bok choy, and cabbage and stir-fry for 3 minutes.

4. Add the edamame, garlic, ginger, and chipotle powder and stir-fry for 2 minutes. Add the tamari and sesame chili oil and stir-fry for 3 minutes, until the vegetables are cooked through. Remove the pan from the heat.

1 cup thinly sliced green cabbage

½ cup shelled thawed edamame

3 large cloves garlic, micro-grated

1½ tablespoons micro-grated peeled fresh ginger

½ teaspoon chipotle powder

¼ cup gluten-free tamari

½ teaspoon sesame chili oil

4 ounces bean sprouts

Juice of 1 large lime

½ cup loosely packed cilantro, chopped

3 tablespoons thinly sliced green onions

1 avocado, pitted, peeled, and sliced

5. Add the rice to the vegetables, return the pan to medium heat, and cook, stirring often, for 5 minutes. Reduce the heat to low and mix in the bean sprouts, 3 tablespoons of the slivered almonds, and the lime juice.

6. Divide the stir-fry among four bowls and top evenly with the remaining 1 tablespoon almonds, the cilantro, green onions, and avocado.

Resistant-Starch Kitchari

Serves: 4

Prep Time: 20 minutes,
plus 1 hour chilling
Cook Time: 1 hour

Beet-Pickled Onions

1 medium red onion, cut
into ⅛-inch-thick slices

1 tablespoon minced peeled
red beet

½ cup apple cider vinegar

½ teaspoon sea salt

5 whole black peppercorns

Resistant-Starch Rice

½ cup white basmati rice,
rinsed until the water
runs clear

2 cups filtered water

1 tablespoon coconut oil

Spice Mixture

1½ teaspoons cumin seed

1½ teaspoons fennel seed

½ teaspoon fenugreek seed

¼ teaspoon yellow
mustard seed

2 teaspoons ground ginger

1½ teaspoons ground
coriander

1½ teaspoons ground garlic

1½ teaspoons ground turmeric

1 teaspoon onion powder

Kitchari, an Indian dish of basmati rice and mung dal (split mung beans), is considered a cleansing and detoxifying dish in Ayurvedic medicine. In this version, white rice is cooked with coconut oil and cooled to create resistant starch—an indigestible starch that doesn't raise blood sugar the way white rice normally does. It also feeds your good gut bacteria. With an aromatic blend of anti-inflammatory spices, mung dal, and vegetables, this recipe gives a whole new meaning to the idea of comfort food.

1. For the pickled onions: Place the onion, beet, vinegar, salt, and peppercorns in a small jar, cover, and let stand for 20 minutes. (This can be done one day in advance. Leftovers will last for up to 2 weeks in the fridge.)

2. For the rice: Combine the rice and water in a medium pot and bring to a boil. Stir in the coconut oil. Cover, reduce the heat to low, and simmer for 20 minutes. Uncover, spread out on a plate, and immediately transfer to the fridge to cool for a minimum of 1 hour.

3. While the rice cools, make the spice mixture: Warm an 8-inch heavy-bottomed skillet over medium-high heat. Add the cumin, fennel, fenugreek, and mustard seeds and cook, shaking the pan often, until the seeds are toasted and begin to "pop." Transfer the mixture to a small bowl and add the ground ginger, coriander, garlic, turmeric, and onion. (This can be done a day in advance and stored in an airtight container.)

4. For the mung beans: Combine the spice mixture, broth, mung beans, and kelp in a medium pot. Cover and simmer, stirring occasionally as the mixture thickens, for 30 minutes.

5. While the mung beans cook, cook the vegetables: Heat a large pot over medium heat and add the coconut oil. Once shimmering, add the carrot, celery, and mushrooms. Stir to combine and sauté for 5 minutes. Add the mung bean mixture to the vegetables, cover, and cook for 20 minutes. Stir in the cooled rice.

Mung Beans and Vegetables

3 cups vegetable broth

½ cup split mung beans
(mung dal)

1 (2-inch) strip kelp

2 tablespoons coconut oil

1 small carrot, finely chopped

1 celery stalk, finely chopped

2 cups cremini mushrooms,
thinly sliced

To Serve

4 large pasture-raised eggs
(optional)

2 teaspoons coconut oil
(optional)

1 avocado, pitted, peeled,
and thinly sliced

½ cup loosely packed fresh
cilantro, roughly chopped

6. If using eggs, melt the coconut oil in a large nonstick pan over medium heat. Crack the eggs into the pan and cook sunny-side-up until the whites are set, about 3 minutes.

7. To serve, split the kitchari among four bowls, topping each with an egg (if you like), drained pickled onions, avocado, and cilantro.

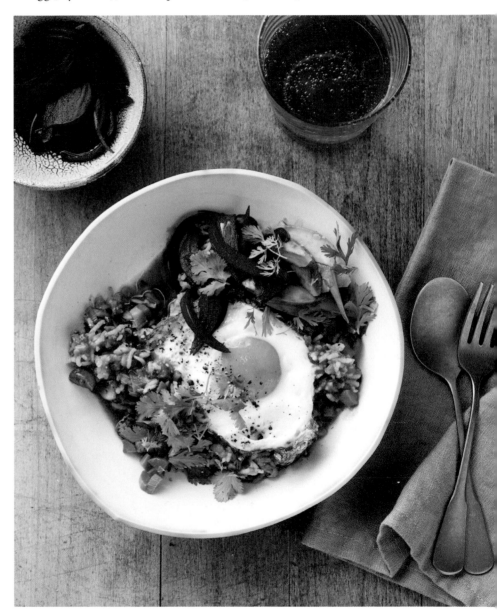

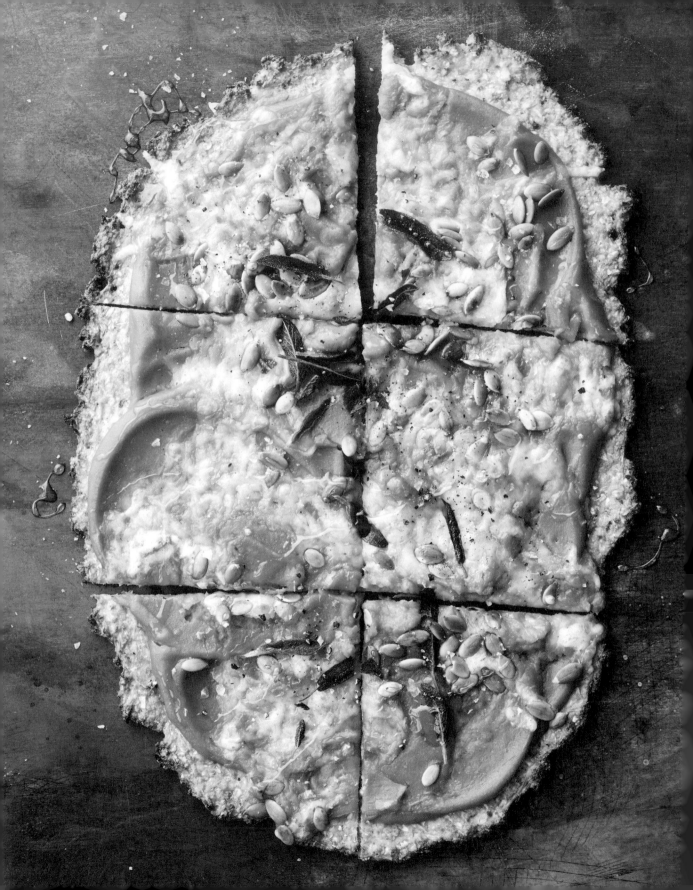

Toasted Sage Butternut Pizza

Cauliflower makes the perfect crust for these delicious pizzas. Topped with a creamy butternut squash sauce, toasted sage, and gooey goat cheese, this is sure to become a new household favorite. It's a much healthier alternative to regular pizza made out of white flour and dairy since it contains a variety of vitamins and minerals and has a lower-glycemic index.

Serves: 4 to 6

Prep Time: 20 minutes
Cook Time: 45 minutes

Butternut Squash Purée

1 small butternut squash (about 1 pound)

2 tablespoons avocado oil

2 tablespoons ghee or coconut oil

3 shallots, chopped

¼ cup chicken broth or filtered water

¼ cup canned coconut cream (unshaken so cream and water are separated)

2 cloves garlic, sliced

Cauliflower Crust

1 medium cauliflower

3 large pasture-raised eggs

1 tablespoon Dijon mustard

1 teaspoon dried oregano

2 teaspoons sea salt

1½ teaspoons freshly ground black pepper

⅔ cup almond flour (or 1 cup chickpea flour)

Toppings

2 tablespoons avocado oil

36 small to medium fresh sage leaves

½ cup grated hard sheep or goat cheese

¼ cup pepitas

1 tablespoon plus 1 teaspoon raw honey (optional)

Pinch of Maldon salt or other flaked salt (optional)

1. To roast the squash for the purée: Preheat the oven to 425°F using a convection setting if possible. Line two baking sheets with parchment paper. Remove the skin from the squash and chop into small cubes. In a baking dish, toss the squash with the avocado oil; roast for 25 minutes or until browned. Keep the oven on.

2. Meanwhile, for the crust: To rice the cauliflower, remove the outer green leaves and most of the stem. Chop the remaining cauliflower into medium chunks and pulse in a food processor until it resembles a fine grain. Alternatively, you can grate the cauliflower on a box grater.

3. Whisk the eggs in a small bowl. Add the cauliflower, mustard, oregano, 1 teaspoon of the salt, and ½ teaspoon of the pepper and mix well. Add the almond flour and mix again. Divide the cauliflower mixture among the two baking sheets, forming 2 oval crusts with hands, ⅛- to ¼-inch thick. Bake the cauliflower crusts for 7 minutes. Remove from the oven, flip the crusts, and rotate the baking sheets between the top and bottom oven racks. Bake for another 8 minutes, until golden, then remove from the oven but keep the oven on.

4. To finish the squash purée: Heat the ghee in a medium pan until shimmering. Add the shallots and sauté 5 minutes. Add the roasted squash, broth, coconut cream, and garlic. Cook for 2 minutes, until hot. Let cool, then purée in a high-speed blender.

5. For the sage topping: Heat the avocado oil in a small pan. Add the sage leaves and cook for 45 seconds, until aromatic and slightly crisp. Remove from the heat.

6. To top the pizzas: Top both crusts with the squash purée, then add the sage leaves, cheese, and pepitas. Bake for 5 minutes, until the cheese is melted. Top the pizzas with the honey and Maldon salt, if desired, and serve.

Lemon-Berry Rose Cream Cake
(page 226)

Desserts

There's no reason the occasional treat can't have a place in a healthy whole-foods diet— the trick is choosing high-quality ingredients. These dessert options taste totally indulgent, but they come with a host of nutrients like good fats, antioxidants, vitamins, and minerals. When it comes to sweeteners, I always recommend sticking with those that are less processed and in their most natural state, like dates, honey, and maple syrup. And of course, a little goes a long way! Enjoy these wholesome treats as part of a mindful approach to eating and a balanced lifestyle.

Cacao–Brazil Nut Bites

Makes: 8 balls

Prep Time: 15 minutes,
plus 30 minutes chilling

½ cup raw Brazil nuts

½ cup unsweetened
shredded coconut

¼ cup raw cacao powder

¼ teaspoon sea salt

½ teaspoon vanilla extract

Large pinch ground cinnamon

2 tablespoons raw honey

These tasty bites are a decadent yet healthy treat thanks to rich, flavorful cacao powder, which is a great source of magnesium and antioxidants. Brazil nuts are less commonly used nuts, but they offer a lot in the way of nutrition, like a generous dose of selenium. This is the perfect quick and easy recipe for satisfying a chocolate craving in a balanced way.

1. Process the nuts and coconut in a food processor until crumbly, then add all the remaining ingredients and pulse a few times to combine.

2. With hands, roll the mixture into 8 small balls, using about 2 tablespoons for each. Place on a large parchment-lined plate or baking sheet without letting them touch.

3. Chill in the freezer for 30 minutes, then enjoy. The chilled balls can be stored in an airtight container in the fridge for up to 1 week, or in the freezer for 2 months.

Cacao-Coconut Custard

Cacao is a powerful superfood—as long as it's not combined with processed sugar and milk. On its own, cacao is a rich source of antioxidants, like anti-inflammatory flavonols and anti-aging polyphenols. Cacao also contains calming magnesium and feel-good plant compounds like anandamide and theobromine that support a focused mind and positive attitude.

Serves: 4

Prep Time: 5 minutes, plus 4 hours chilling

1 can full-fat unsweetened coconut milk

½ cup Medjool dates, pitted and chopped

¼ cup raw cacao powder

½ teaspoon ground cinnamon

Sea salt

¼ cup chia seeds

4 teaspoons cacao nibs

1. Combine the coconut milk, dates, cacao powder, cinnamon, and a pinch of salt in a blender or food processor. Blend until frothy, about 1 minute.

2. In a medium bowl, combine the coconut milk mixture with chia seeds and stir until combined. Taste and add more salt if desired. Cover and chill in the fridge for 4 hours or overnight.

3. To serve, spoon the custard into four small bowls and top each with 1 teaspoon cacao nibs.

Chocolate Caramel Almond-Butter Cups

Makes: 12 cups

Prep Time: 20 minutes, plus 10 minutes chilling

Cook Time: 2 minutes

Chocolate

¾ cup plus 2 tablespoons coconut oil

¾ cup raw cacao powder

⅓ cup plus 1 teaspoon maple syrup

¼ teaspoon sea salt

Caramel Filling

5 pitted Medjool dates, soaked in very hot water for 10 minutes

1 tablespoon almond butter

1 teaspoon almond milk

¼ teaspoon vanilla extract

Almond Butter Filling

¼ cup almond butter

1½ teaspoons maple syrup

1 teaspoon ashwagandha powder

These creamy, decadent chocolate and nut butter cups will leave you feeling calm and relaxed, thanks to all the magnesium and feel-good chemicals found in cacao, along with the mood-balancing effects of the adaptogenic herb ashwagandha. Dates blended into caramel create an extra layer of indulgent filling. I love having a few of these in the freezer at all times for a quick dessert or occasional midday pick-me-up.

1. Line 12 muffin cups with paper liners.

2. For the chocolate: In a small pot over low heat, melt together the coconut oil, cacao powder, maple syrup, and salt, about 2 minutes. Remove from the heat. Spoon 2 teaspoons of the chocolate into each lined muffin cup, then transfer the cups to the freezer to harden, about 5 minutes. Set the remaining chocolate aside.

3. For the caramel filling: Drain the dates well and mince. In a small bowl, stir together the almond butter, almond milk, and vanilla. Stir in the dates and mix thoroughly. Set aside.

4. For the almond butter filling: Mix together the almond butter, maple syrup, and ashwagandha in a small bowl. Scoop out twelve 1½-teaspoon portions, place on a piece of parchment paper, and form into little pucks slightly smaller than the base of the muffin liners.

5. Place an almond butter puck on top of the chocolate base inside each muffin cup, making sure the puck doesn't touch the side of the liner. Top each with ½ teaspoon of the caramel filling. Spoon the remaining chocolate over the filling, 4 teaspoons per muffin cup.

6. Place the cups in the freezer to harden, about 10 minutes, then enjoy. Store almond butter cups in an airtight container in the fridge or freezer for up to 1 month.

Salted Pecan-Fudge Cookies

Cookies are just one of those classic comfort foods. This recipe makes a grain-free, dairy-free fudgy cookie with a delightful hint of pecan and sea salt. Chocolate and pecans are both incredible sources of antioxidants, and almond flour is a great alternative to white flour, providing more protein, fiber, and nutrients like vitamin E without producing the same rise in blood sugar.

Makes: 12 cookies

Prep Time: 20 minutes, plus 10 minutes chilling

Cook Time: 15 minutes

1 cup pecan butter or almond butter

½ cup coconut oil (not melted)

½ cup coconut sugar

2 large pasture-raised eggs

1 teaspoon vanilla extract

½ cup almond flour

½ teaspoon ground cinnamon (optional)

½ teaspoon sea salt

6 ounces dark chocolate (70 percent or more cacao), shaved and chopped

½ cup raw pecans, chopped

1 teaspoon Maldon sea salt flakes

1. Preheat the oven to 350°F; line two baking sheets with parchment paper.

2. Using a hand or stand mixer, cream the nut butter, coconut oil, sugar, eggs, and vanilla together in a large bowl. In a medium bowl, combine the almond flour, cinnamon (if using), salt, chocolate, and pecans. Add to the nut butter mixture, stirring well by hand. Place the dough in the freezer for 10 minutes before baking.

3. When ready, scoop 2-tablespoon portions of dough onto the lined baking sheets, leaving adequate space between each. Crumble large sea salt flakes in your hand and sprinkle evenly over the tops of the cookies.

4. Bake for 15 minutes, rotating pans between the oven racks halfway through. Cookies will be soft when removed from the oven but will firm as they cool. Let cool on trays several minutes before moving to a cooling rack.

Chocolate-Almond Sandwich Cookies

Crunchy, creamy, buttery, and chocolatey—these cookies are an unbelievable treat. A luscious chocolate filling with a hint of maple is layered between two spiced almond cookies. They will melt in your mouth. Enjoy them with a cold glass of my Spiced Brazil Nut Milk (page 243).

Makes: 10 sandwich cookies

Prep Time: 20 minutes, plus 30 minutes chilling
Cook Time: 12 to 14 minutes

Cookies

2½ cups fine almond flour

½ cup arrowroot or kudzu root powder

2 tablespoons coconut flour

1 teaspoon baking soda

2 teaspoons ground cinnamon

½ teaspoon grated nutmeg

½ teaspoon sea salt

¼ cup ghee or coconut oil, melted

½ cup maple syrup or coconut nectar

1 teaspoon vanilla extract

Chocolate Filling

8 ounces unsalted butter or coconut oil, at room temperature

3 tablespoons raw cacao powder

2 tablespoons maple syrup (optional)

1. For the cookies: In a large bowl, combine the almond flour, arrowroot, coconut flour, baking soda, cinnamon, nutmeg, and salt. Stir in the melted ghee, maple syrup, and vanilla, then mix until well combined and able to form a ball.

2. Divide the dough in two. Wrap each half in parchment paper, tightening the sides and shaping to form two long, even logs, about 4 inches long and 2 inches in diameter. Place in the fridge to solidify for a minimum of 30 minutes, or up to 1 day.

3. When ready to bake, preheat the oven to 350°F; line two baking sheets with parchment paper.

4. Remove the dough from the parchment and slice each log into ten rounds. Place the dough rounds on the lined baking sheets, spaced evenly to allow room to spread. Bake for 6 minutes. Rotate the baking sheets between the top and bottom oven racks and bake for another 6 to 8 minutes, until the cookies are golden. Let cool on a wire rack. The cookies will crisp up as they cool.

5. For the filling: While the cookies bake, beat the room temperature butter with the cacao and maple syrup.

6. Once the cookies have cooled, make sandwiches by spreading 1 heaping tablespoon filling onto half the cookies, then top each with another cookie. Serve immediately. To prepare ahead of time, store the cookies in an airtight container on the countertop and refrigerate the filling, covered; assemble just prior to serving.

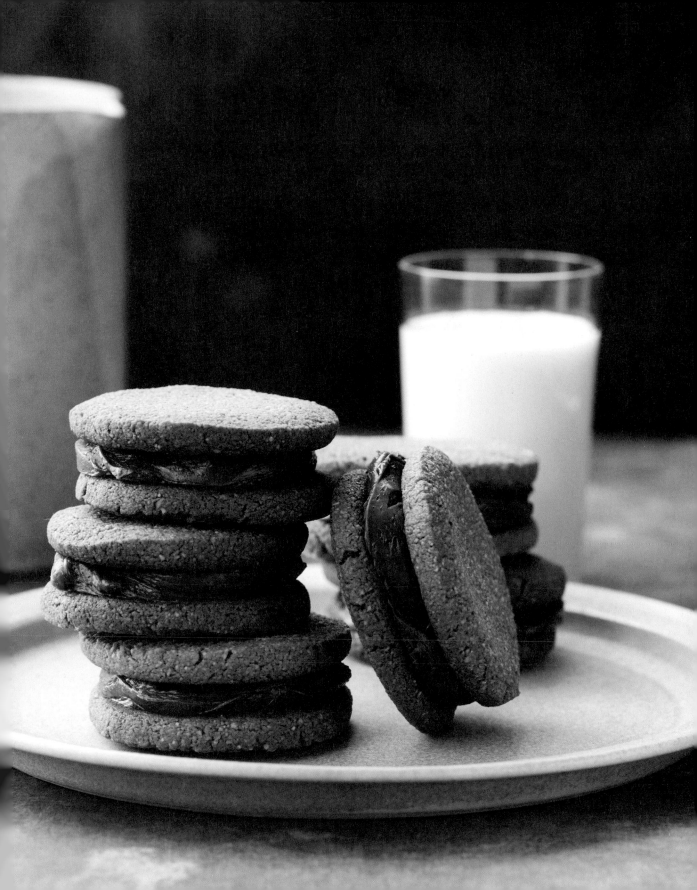

Lemon-Berry Rose Cream Cake

Serves: 16

Prep Time: 30 minutes, plus 3 hours soaking and 2 hours chilling

Crust

2 cups raw walnuts

½ cup raw almonds

1 cup tightly packed Medjool dates, pitted, chopped, plus more if needed

3 tablespoons coconut oil, melted

Large pinch of sea salt

White Filling

3½ cups raw cashews, soaked in water at least 3 hours or overnight

¾ cup fresh lemon juice (about 4 large lemons)

½ cup canned coconut cream (unshaken so cream and water are separated)

½ cup coconut water (from the can of coconut cream)

¼ cup blonde coconut nectar

1 tablespoon coconut oil, melted

2½ teaspoons vanilla extract

1 teaspoon food-grade rose water, or more to taste

This show-stopping cake is as unique and tasty as it sounds, and it requires no cooking at all! Cashews blend into a silky dairy-free cream, creating the perfect base for the flavors of fresh lemon juice, tangy raspberries, and a hint of rose. Rose water potency can vary by brand, so taste as you go and adjust to your liking. Two layers of smooth filling over a crumbly walnut crust create the perfect bite—this cake never lasts long!

1. Line the bottom of a 9-inch springform pan with parchment paper.

2. For the crust: Combine the walnuts and almonds in a food processor and blend well. Add the chopped dates, coconut oil, and salt and blend until mixed into a fine crumb. It should be crumbly but sticky when pressed together; add an extra date if needed. Using your hands, press this mix into the bottom of the pan, making sure to spread it evenly and flat.

3. For the white filling: Drain the cashews and rinse with cold water. Combine the cashews, lemon juice, coconut cream, coconut water, coconut nectar, melted coconut oil, vanilla, and rose water in a high-speed blender. Blend on low and slowly increase to high. Stop to scrape the sides as needed and continue blending until super smooth.

4. Scoop 2½ cups of the filling into the crust and spread evenly with the back of a spoon. Leave the extra filling in the blender. Place the crust in the freezer.

5. For the pink filling layer: Add the coconut cream, coconut oil, rose water, and raspberries to the blender with the remaining white filling. Blend well, increasing speed from low to high until everything is fully incorporated and no lumps remain. Pour the pink filling on top of the white layer. Again, use a spoon to spread evenly. Return to the freezer and freeze for at least 2 hours.

6. Remove the cake from the freezer and garnish with berries, shredded coconut, and lemon zest. Let thaw 5 to 10 minutes before slicing; thawing time will depend on how long the cake was in the freezer. For an ice cream texture, serve soon after slicing; for a cheesecake texture, let thaw an additional 10 minutes after slicing.

Pink Filling

2 tablespoons canned coconut cream

1 tablespoon coconut oil, melted

½ teaspoon food-grade rose water, or more to taste

6 ounces fresh raspberries

Garnish

Fresh raspberries, blueberries, blackberries, and quartered strawberries

1 teaspoon unsweetened shredded coconut

½ teaspoon lemon zest

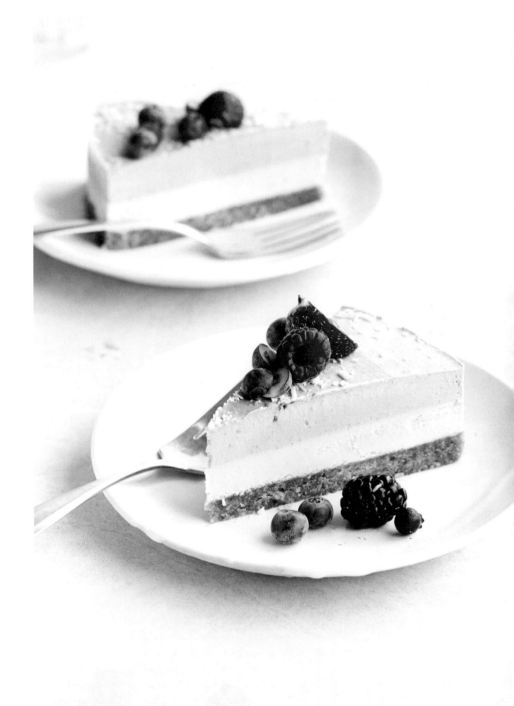

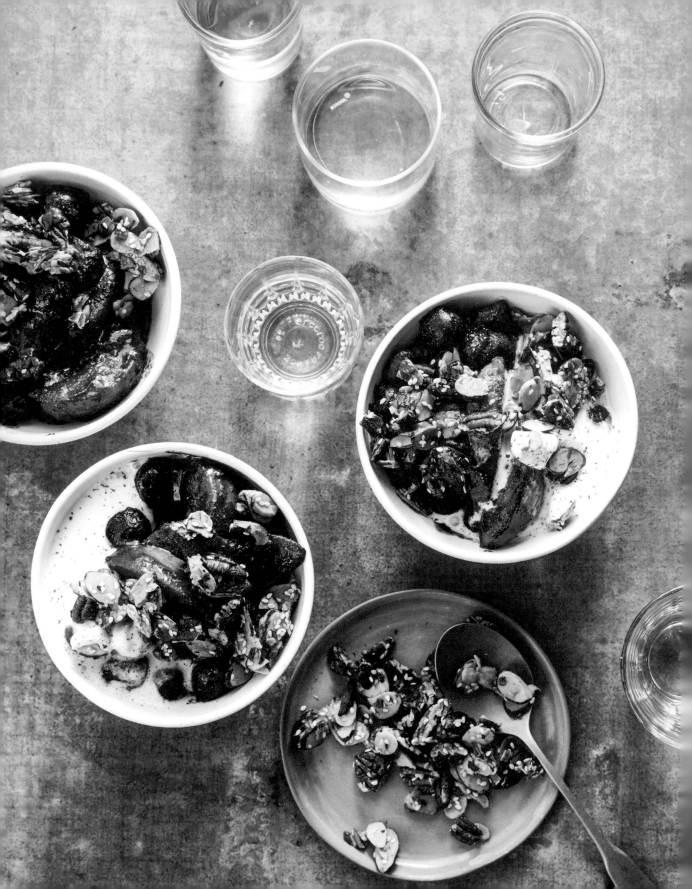

Maple Harvest Crisp

Serves: 8

Prep Time: 10 minutes
Cook Time: 40 minutes

1 (12-ounce) bag frozen peaches

2 (12-ounce) bags frozen cherries

¼ cup almond flour

1½ tablespoons ground flaxseed

1 teaspoon ground cinnamon, plus more for garnish

1½ cups raw sliced almonds

1 cup raw pecans, chopped

2 tablespoons white sesame seeds

2 tablespoons maple syrup

1½ teaspoons coconut oil, melted

¼ teaspoon sea salt

½ cup canned coconut cream (unshaken so cream and water are separated)

Gooey baked peaches and cherries topped with an incredibly crunchy, sweet, and salty granola—it's as amazing as it sounds. This fruit-filled crisp is full of antioxidants, anti-inflammatory phytonutrients, and fiber, so you can enjoy a treat without compromising your health. A dollop of coconut cream brings it all together and adds a dose of satiating, beneficial fats.

1. Preheat the oven to 375°F. Grease an 8x8-inch baking dish and line a baking sheet with parchment paper.

2. In a large bowl, combine the peaches, cherries, almond flour, flaxseed, and cinnamon. Stir well until the fruit is coated. Transfer to the greased baking dish and bake for 30 minutes.

3. In a medium bowl, make the granola by mixing together the almonds, pecans, sesame seeds, maple syrup, coconut oil, and salt until well combined. Pour the mixture onto the lined baking sheet, spreading evenly but keeping some parts clustered.

4. After the fruit has baked for 30 minutes, put the granola in the oven. Bake both, separately, for 10 minutes, until the granola is golden and slightly crispy; it will crisp more as it cools. Remove the granola from the oven and set aside to cool. Then check on the fruit—it will be hot in the center and bubbling around the edges when ready. Bake for an additional 5 minutes if needed.

5. To serve, top the fruit evenly with the granola. Portion into individual bowls and top with the coconut cream and a dash of cinnamon.

Maple Pumpkin Pie

CONTRIBUTED BY DANIELLE WALKER

Serves: 8 to 10

Prep Time: 30 minutes, plus 3¾ hours cooling and chilling

Cook Time: 1 hour 5 minutes

Basic Pie Pastry

2½ cups blanched almond flour

1 cup arrowroot powder

¼ cup coconut sugar

2 large pasture-raised eggs, chilled

3 tablespoons cold filtered water

½ teaspoon fine sea salt

¼ cup coconut oil or butter (not melted)

Egg wash of 1 large pasture-raised egg yolk beaten with 1 tablespoon full-fat unsweetened coconut milk

Pumpkin Filling

2 cups fresh pumpkin purée, or 1 (15-ounce) can puréed pumpkin

3 large pasture-raised eggs

½ cup full-fat unsweetened coconut milk

This amazing pumpkin pie comes from one of my favorite cookbook authors and food bloggers, Danielle Walker of Against All Grain. It's the perfect ending to any fall or winter meal, but without the grains, dairy, and refined sugar found in traditional pies.

1. For the pie pastry: Combine the almond flour, arrowroot, coconut sugar, eggs, water, and salt in a food processor. Process for 10 seconds, or until combined. Add the coconut oil, distributing 1 tablespoon at a time evenly over the dough. Pulse four or five times, until pea-size bits of dough form. Gather the dough into a tight ball and flatten into a disk. Wrap tightly and freeze for 1 hour.

2. Preheat the oven to 325°F; line a baking sheet with parchment paper.

3. Reserve one-fourth of the dough for the decorative toppings. Press the remaining dough into the bottom and up the sides of a 9-inch pie plate, using the palms of your hands to ensure the crust is even throughout. Press together any breaks in the dough, then crimp or flute the edges with your fingers. Cut a round of parchment paper to fit the bottom of the crust, place in the crust, and fill with pie weights or dried beans. Freeze until firm, about 15 minutes.

4. Bake the pie crust for 10 minutes. Remove the weights and parchment paper and bake for 5 minutes longer, until the crust is golden. Cool completely on a wire rack.

5. For the decorative pastry: Roll out the reserved pie pastry between two sheets of parchment paper. Use cookie cutters to cut out shapes. Brush the egg wash onto the pastry shapes. Reserve the remaining egg wash. Transfer the shapes to the prepared baking sheet and bake for 15 minutes, until golden. Cool completely on a wire rack.

½ cup pure maple syrup or light-colored raw honey

1 teaspoon ground cinnamon

½ teaspoon ground ginger

½ teaspoon ground nutmeg

¼ teaspoon ground cloves

¼ teaspoon ground cardamom

½ teaspoon finely grated lemon zest

1 teaspoon pure vanilla extract

¼ teaspoon kosher salt

Garnish

Whipped coconut cream

6. Increase the oven temperature to 350°F. Place the pie crust on a rimmed baking sheet and brush the top edge with egg wash.

7. For the filling: Whisk together all the ingredients in a large bowl. Pour the filling into the prepared pie shell and bake for 15 minutes. Cover the edge of the crust with foil and continue baking for 20 minutes, until the custard has set but still jiggles slightly in the center. Leave the pie in the oven, turn off the oven, and leave the door cracked open for 30 minutes while the pie cools.

8. Remove the pie from the oven and let cool to room temperature on a wire rack. Place the decorative pastry cutouts around the perimeter of the pie. Refrigerate until fully set, about 2 hours. Serve with whipped coconut cream.

Reprinted with permission from Danielle Walker's *Against All Grain Celebrations.*

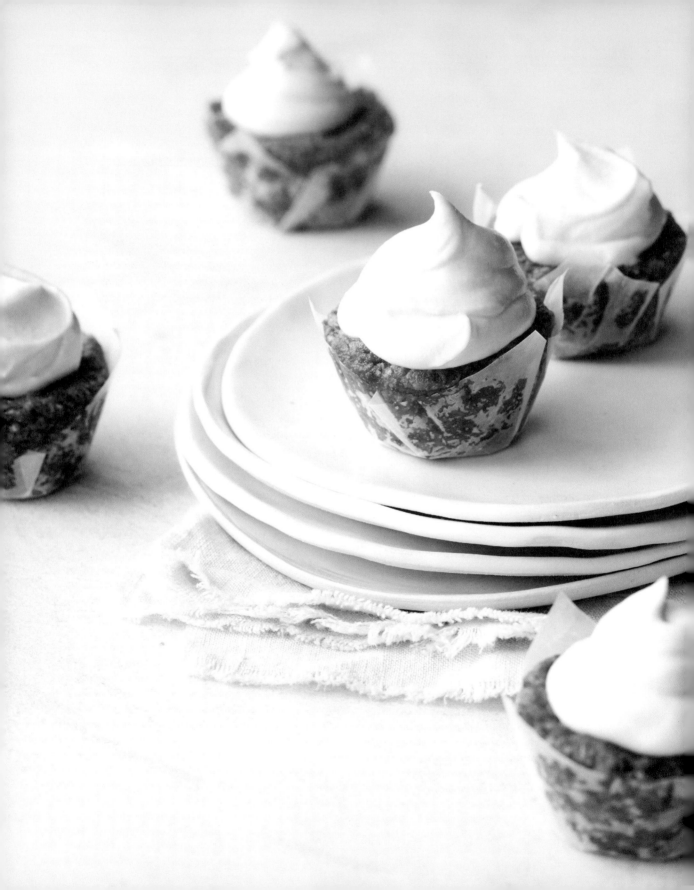

No-Bake Carrot Mini Cupcakes with Honey Vanilla Buttercream

Makes: 12 mini cupcakes

Prep Time: 20 minutes, plus 3 hours soaking and 30 minutes chilling

Honey Vanilla "Buttercream"

¼ cup plus 2 tablespoons raw cashews

Juice of ½ lemon

2 tablespoons canned coconut cream (unshaken so cream and water are separated)

1½ tablespoons raw honey

1½ teaspoons coconut oil, soft but not melted

¼ teaspoon vanilla extract

Cupcakes

1⅓ cups raw walnuts

8 Medjool dates, pitted, chopped, plus more if needed

⅔ cup unsweetened shredded coconut

3 tablespoons coconut oil

1¼ teaspoons ground cinnamon

¾ teaspoon ground ginger

¼ teaspoon ground cardamom

¼ teaspoon ground nutmeg

¼ teaspoon sea salt

1⅓ cups finely grated carrots, patted dry

A healthy spin on a classic treat, these cute cupcakes are perfectly spiced and topped with a rich, dairy-free "buttercream" made from blended cashews—without all the refined sugar and flour found in traditional carrot cake. Carrots are a great source of beta-carotene and dates are rich in potassium and magnesium, so you can enjoy dessert and get some beneficial nutrients while you're at it.

1. For the buttercream: Soak the cashews in water at least 3 hours or overnight. Rinse with cold water and drain well. Combine the cashews, lemon juice, coconut cream, honey, coconut oil, and vanilla in a blender and begin blending on low. Slowly increase the speed until smooth and creamy, stopping to scrape down sides as needed. Pour into a bowl, cover, and refrigerate while you work on the cupcakes.

2. For the cupcakes: Pulse the walnuts, dates, shredded coconut, coconut oil, cinnamon, ginger, cardamom, nutmeg, and salt in a food processor until the mixture holds together, about 3 minutes. If needed, add an extra date to help the mixture stick. Fold in the carrots by hand and combine well.

3. Line a 12-cup mini muffin pan with paper liners. Using 2 tablespoons per cupcake, scoop the batter into the liners and press firmly with fingers. Use a spoon to place a dollop of buttercream on each cupcake. Chill the cupcakes in the fridge for at least 30 minutes before serving.

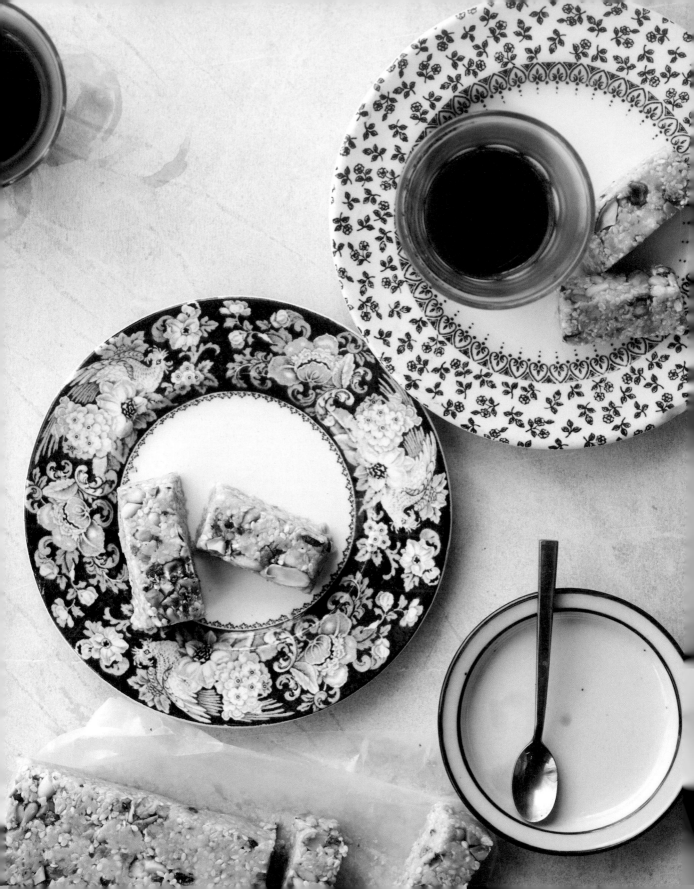

Turkish Halva

Halva is a delectable Middle Eastern treat made with sesame paste and seeds. I add fiber-rich almond flour and antioxidant-rich pistachios and use date nectar as a cleaner sweetener option—you could also use honey. A little taste of these rich bites goes a long way!

Makes: 16 to 18 pieces

Prep Time: 5 minutes, plus 1 hour chilling

Cook Time: 3 minutes

¼ cup raw pine nuts

½ cup almond flour

½ cup tahini

½ cup sesame seeds

¼ cup unsweetened shredded coconut

¼ cup date nectar or 3 tablespoons raw honey

½ teaspoon vanilla extract

¼ cup raw pistachios

1. Heat a small sauté pan over medium-high heat. Add the pine nuts and stir frequently until fragrant and toasted, about 3 minutes. Remove from the heat and set aside.

2. In a medium bowl, mix together the almond flour, tahini, sesame seeds, coconut, date nectar, and vanilla. Mix with a wooden spoon or a spatula until all the ingredients are combined.

3. In a food processor, pulse the toasted pine nuts and the pistachios until crushed. Fold the nuts into the tahini mixture. Pour the mixture into a greased 8½ x 4½-inch loaf pan, spreading evenly and tapping the pan on the counter to release bubbles. Refrigerate for a minimum of 1 hour. When ready to serve, slice into bite-size pieces and enjoy.

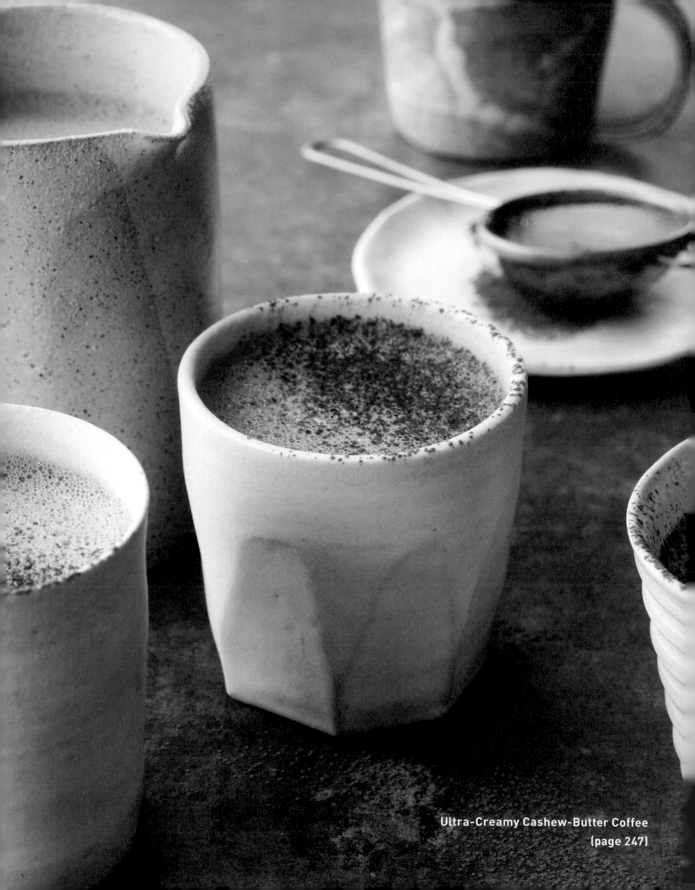

Ultra-Creamy Cashew-Butter Coffee
(page 247)

Beverages

Staying hydrated is an essential part of feeling great. It lubricates your joints, keeps skin looking young, supports a healthy brain, helps the body eliminate toxins, and so much more. Many of the unique beverages in this section will hydrate you; others provide a variety of other health benefits thanks to functional ingredients like turmeric, mint, and medicinal mushrooms.

Medicinal Mushroom Tonic

Serves: 2

Prep Time: 5 minutes

6 (1,000-milligram) medicinal mushroom capsules (chaga, lion's mane, reishi, turkey tail, cordyceps, etc.)

2 cups unsweetened coconut or almond milk

1 tablespoon MCT oil

1 teaspoon vanilla extract

½ teaspoon ground cinnamon

1 tablespoon maple syrup (optional)

Mushrooms are one of nature's many amazing medicines. You can tailor the medicinal mushrooms in this frothy drink to meet your own health needs—use chaga for an immune boost, cordyceps for anti-inflammatory and antioxidant benefits, or lion's mane for extra focus and productivity. All of these options provide multiple health benefits and different subtle flavors, so get creative and see what you can blend up!

1. Open the mushroom capsules and pour the powder into a small bowl.

2. Gently warm the milk in a saucepan over medium heat, 4 to 5 minutes. Pour into a blender and add the mushroom powder and the remaining ingredients. Blend on high until frothy, about 45 seconds. Drink immediately.

Uplifting Herbal Hemp Latte

Serves: 1

Prep Time: 5 minutes

1½ cups hot filtered water

3 tablespoons hemp seeds

1 large Medjool date, pitted

1 teaspoon ashwagandha powder

1 teaspoon MCT oil

¼ teaspoon ground cinnamon

Pinch of ground nutmeg

Pinch of sea salt

Ashwagandha is an adaptogen, a type of herb that nourishes the adrenal glands and helps your body better adapt to stress. It can also support healthy thyroid hormones and balanced blood sugar. With all these benefits, this latte makes a warm and comforting drink, perfect for a cold day.

1. Combine all ingredients in a blender and blend until smooth. Drink right away.

Sparkling Emerald Tea

Serves: 4

Prep Time: 5 minutes, plus 20 minutes steeping and 2 hours chilling

6 cups filtered water

6 peppermint tea bags

2 limes, halved

1 teaspoon apple cider vinegar

2 teaspoons mint-flavored liquid chlorophyll

1 cup sparkling mineral water

Fresh mint

Chlorophyll is the green pigment found in plants that helps them turn light into energy. In humans, it can improve detoxification, slow or prevent cancer growth, and possibly support stronger red blood cells. Peppermint is helpful for soothing the digestive system and has anti-inflammatory, antibacterial, and antiviral properties. Enjoy this drink any time of day for a refreshing boost.

1. Bring the water to a boil in a saucepan. Once boiling, remove from the heat and add the tea bags. Let steep for 20 minutes. Remove the tea bags and let the tea cool for a minimum of 2 hours.

2. For each serving, combine 1½ cups tea, juice of ½ lime, ¼ teaspoon apple cider vinegar, ½ teaspoon chlorophyll, and ¼ cup sparkling water and serve over ice in an 8-ounce glass. Garnish with mint leaves.

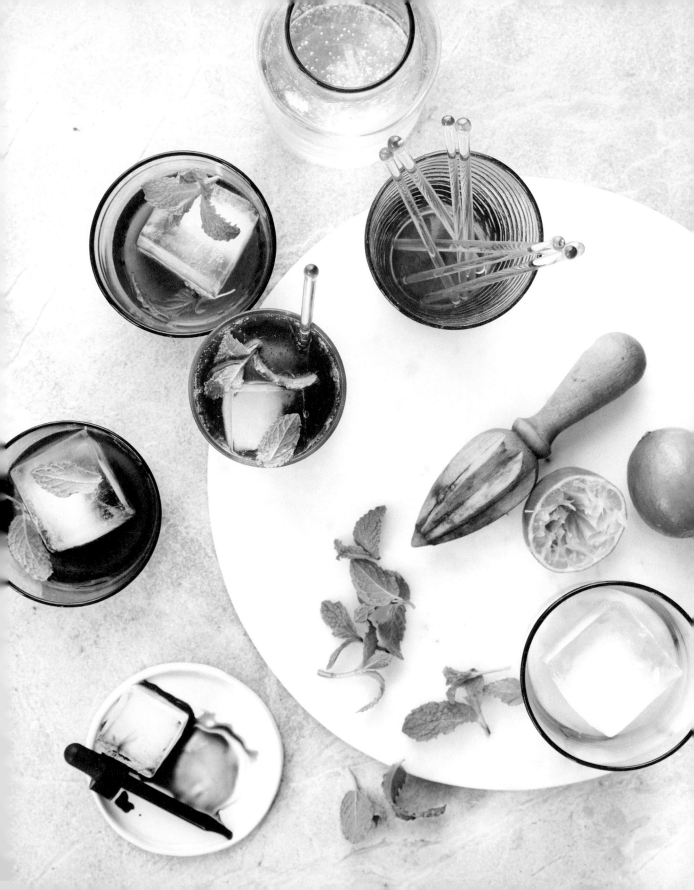

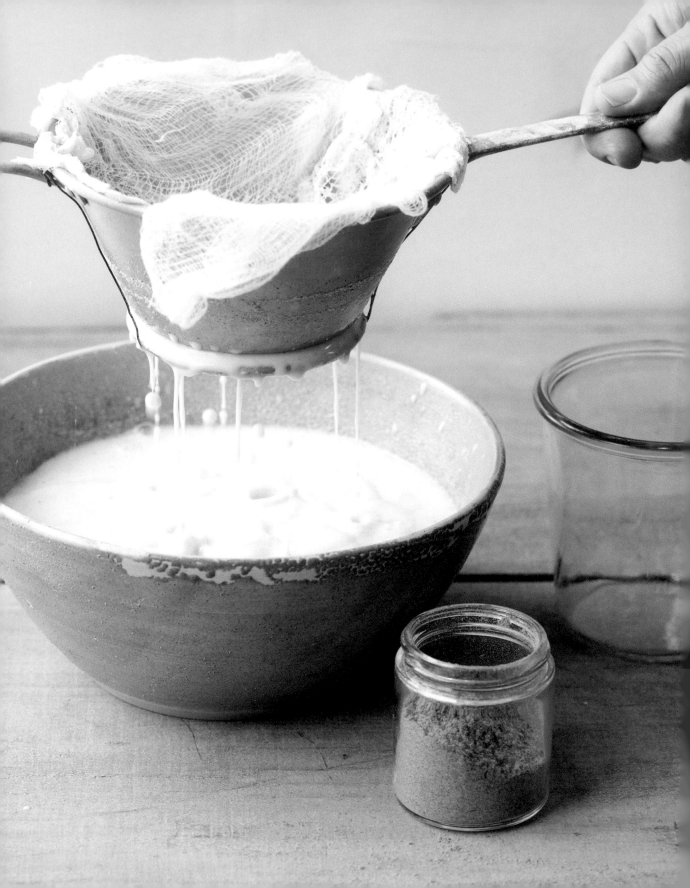

Spiced Brazil Nut Milk

Makes: 4 cups

Prep Time: 5 minutes

4 cups filtered water

2 cups raw Brazil nuts

1¼ teaspoons vanilla extract

½ teaspoon sea salt

¼ teaspoon cardamom powder

Making your own nut milk is incredibly easy. This Brazil nut milk, a tasty homemade alternative to store-bought dairy-free milks, is especially rich in immune-boosting selenium. Sea salt brings out the natural sweetness in the milk while adding extra trace minerals.

1. Combine all the ingredients in a high-speed blender and blend until smooth. Strain through cheesecloth into a large glass jar. Store in the fridge for up to 5 days.

Turmeric Collagen Elixir

Makes: 2 glasses or
4 shots

Prep Time: 5 minutes

2 cups filtered water

¼ cup chopped peeled
fresh ginger

¼ cup chopped peeled
fresh turmeric

1 whole lemon, peeled

Pinch of cayenne

Pinch of freshly ground
black pepper

2 scoops (2 tablespoons)
collagen powder

Turmeric is an amazingly powerful spice—it's anti-inflammatory, antioxidant, and can even increase something called brain-derived neurotrophic factor, which boosts brain function. Collagen adds another healing component for connective tissue, so this elixir supports the brain, gut, skin, and joints all at once. It's a wonderful drink to start the day with so you can feel on point and ready for anything.

1. Combine 1 cup of the water, the ginger, turmeric, lemon, cayenne, and black pepper in a high-speed blender and blend until smooth. Strain through a cheesecloth into a large wide-mouth jar or bowl.

2. Pour the contents back into the blender and add the collagen powder and remaining 1 cup water. Blend well.

3. Consume as a shot, a warm beverage, or pour over ice to enjoy cold.

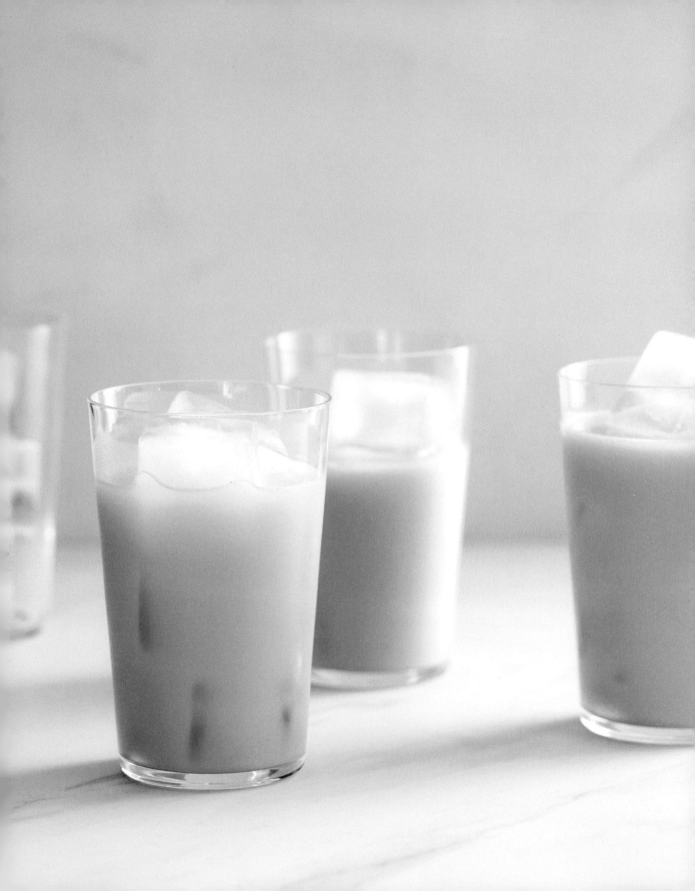

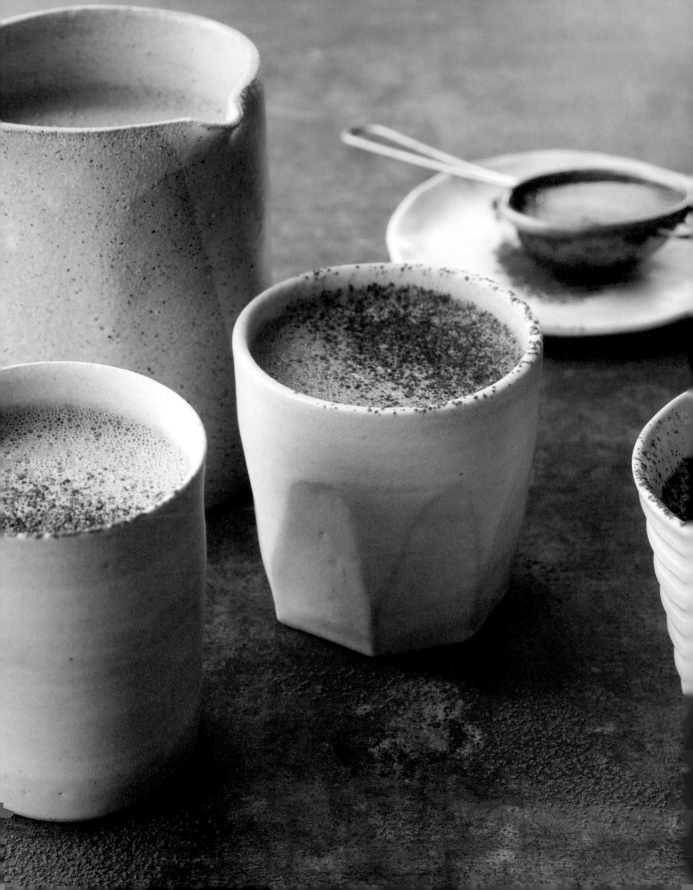

Ultra-Creamy
Cashew-Butter Coffee

Serves: 1

Prep Time: 5 minutes

1 cup coffee (regular or decaf)

2 tablespoons cashew butter

1 tablespoon full-fat
unsweetened coconut milk

2 teaspoons hazelnut extract
(optional)

Pinch of sea salt

Pinch of raw cacao powder

I love to kick off my morning with this energizing blended coffee. Cashew butter is rich in minerals and heart-healthy mono-unsaturated fats. These fats, in combination with the medium-chain triglycerides found in coconut milk, give this drink an ultra-creamy texture and help to balance the effects of caffeine, keeping you focused and alert all morning long.

1. Combine the coffee, cashew butter, coconut milk, hazelnut extract (if using), and salt in a blender and blend until smooth. Pour into a mug and garnish with a sprinkle of cacao powder. Can be enjoyed warm or over ice.

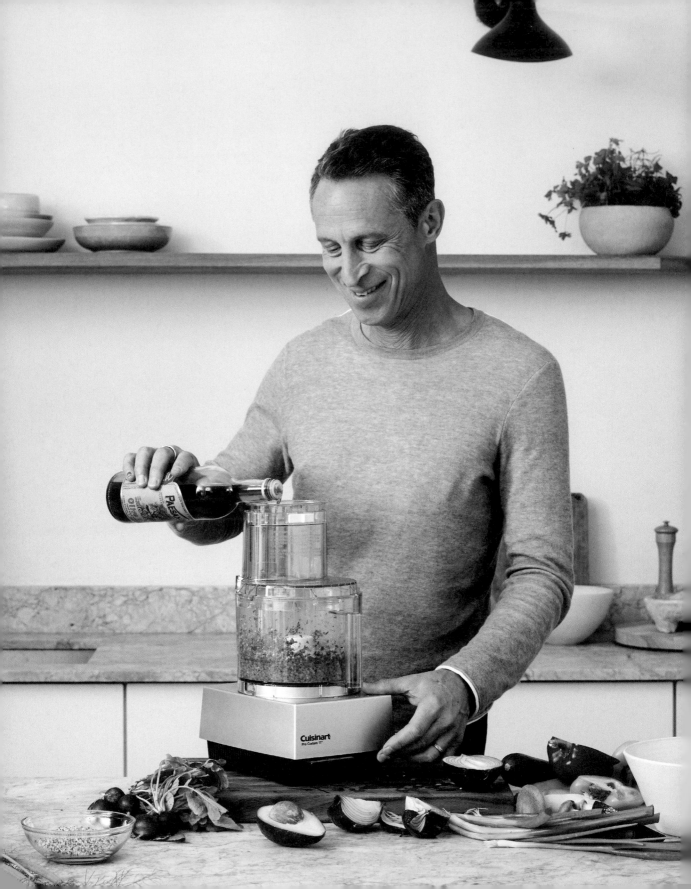

Better Basics

When it comes to clean cooking, it's always important to look at the basics. If your ingredients aren't high-quality, your final dish won't be either. You can easily create simple yet nutritious spice mixes, sauces, dressings, broths, and even bread and crackers to use throughout the rest of your meals. Then you can stock your fridge, freezer, and pantry to be ready for confident cooking.

Avocado Mayo

Makes: 1½ cups

Prep Time: 10 minutes

2 large pasture-raised
egg yolks

1 tablespoon lemon juice

2 teaspoons brown mustard

1 teaspoon sea salt

1½ cups avocado oil

Mayonnaise can be a healthy, go-to condiment—but only if it contains the right kind of oil. Most store-bought varieties include canola oil or other inflammatory fats, but not this version. My homemade mayo uses avocado oil, which provides oleic acid that supports heart health and lutein, an antioxidant that benefits eyesight. Keep a jar on hand so you can easily add a dollop of tangy flavor to your favorite dishes.

1. Place the egg yolks, lemon juice, mustard, and salt in a food processor and blend well.

2. While the machine is running, add the avocado oil very slowly, a few drops at a time. Once the mixture starts to thicken, add the remaining oil in a very slow, thin stream until fully incorporated.

3. Store the mayo in an airtight container in the refrigerator and consume within 1 week.

Chicken Bone Broth

CONTRIBUTED BY CHEF MARCO CANORA

Makes: 6 quarts

Prep Time: 5 minutes

Cook Time: 5½ to
7½ hours

10 pounds chicken necks and
backs (if available, substitute
1 to 2 pounds with chicken feet)

1 (28-ounce) can whole
peeled tomatoes

3 large yellow onions,
coarsely chopped

2 large carrots, scrubbed
and coarsely chopped

6 celery stalks, coarsely
chopped

1 bunch fresh flat-leaf parsley

5 bay leaves

Fine sea salt

1 tablespoon black
peppercorns

This rich, caramelized broth comes from my friend Marco Canora, chef and founder of New York City's Brodo broth shop. You can bring the gut-healing, nourishing properties of his broth into your own kitchen with this amazing recipe. It makes a large pot, so you'll have plenty of leftovers ready to warm and sip as needed.

1. Preheat the oven to 375°F.

2. Arrange the bones in a single layer on rimmed baking sheets (if using chicken feet, set them aside). Roast the bones for about 1 hour, flipping after 30 minutes, until well browned.

3. Put the roasted bones and the feet (if using) in a 16-quart pot. Add enough cold water to cover by 2 to 3 inches. Bring to a boil over high heat. Reduce the heat to low and pull the pot to one side so it is partially off the burner. Simmer for 1 hour and 30 minutes, skimming the top layer of foam every 15 to 20 minutes, as needed.

4. Add the tomatoes, onions, carrots, celery, parsley, bay leaves, salt to taste, and peppercorns and push the ingredients down into the liquid. Continue to simmer for 3 to 5 hours, skimming as needed and occasionally checking to make sure the bones are still fully submerged.

5. Use a spider skimmer or slotted spoon to remove the solids from the broth and discard. Strain the broth through a fine-mesh strainer into a bowl. Season with salt to taste and let cool.

6. Transfer the cooled broth to storage containers (leaving any sediment in the bottom of the bowl) and refrigerate overnight. When the broth is chilled, spoon off any solidified fat. Store the broth in the refrigerator for up to 5 days or in the freezer for up to 6 months.

Cajun Spice Blend

This savory blend is an easy way to spice up any type of meal, from seafood to poultry to a veggie medley. Chili powder, cayenne, and garlic give the mix a zesty kick, and they come along with a great boost for the circulatory system. Oregano and thyme provide a nice contrast with smoother herbaceous flavors.

Makes: 1 cup

Prep Time: 5 minutes

Cook Time: 5 minutes

3 tablespoons garlic powder

2 tablespoons chili powder

2 tablespoons paprika

2 tablespoons onion powder

2 tablespoons dried oregano

1 tablespoon dried thyme

1½ teaspoons cayenne powder

1½ teaspoons smoked paprika

1½ teaspoons coriander powder

1½ tablespoons sea salt

1 tablespoon white pepper

1. Mix all ingredients in a small jar and store in an airtight container for up to 1 year.

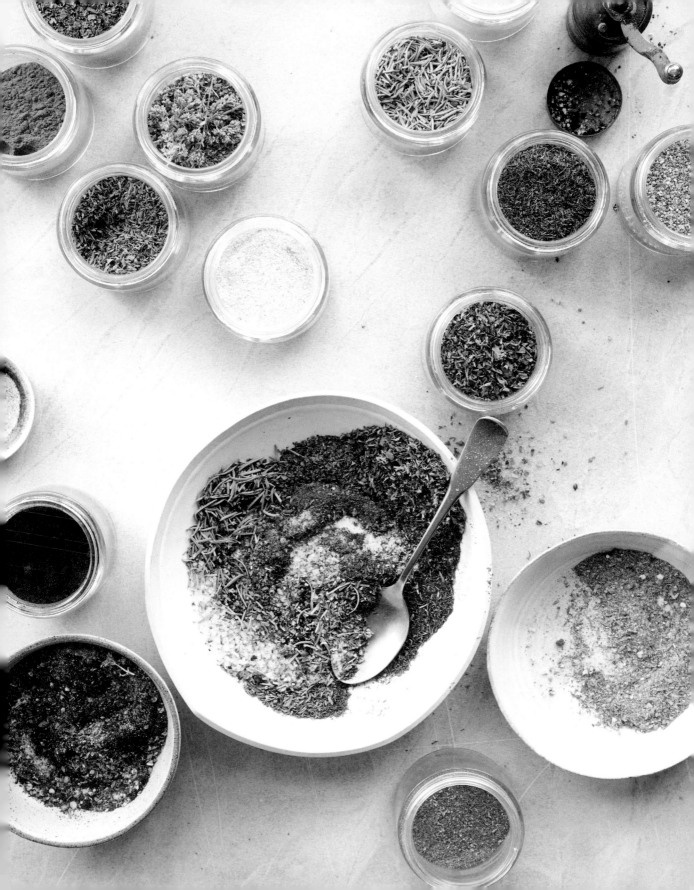

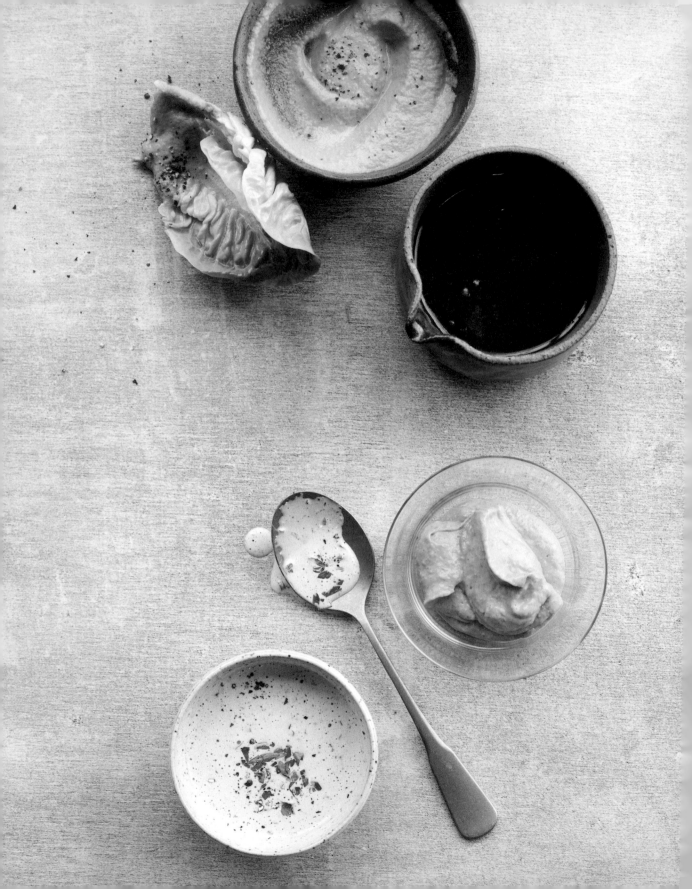

Carrot Ginger Dressing

Making your own dressing at home is an easy way to make a big impact on your diet. This beautiful orange dressing comes together in just a few minutes and is packed with flavor as well as nutrients like beta-carotene and monounsaturated fats. Use on a variety of salads, roasted veggies, and even protein dishes.

Makes: 2 cups

Prep Time: 5 minutes

1 large carrot, peeled and finely chopped (1 cup)

¼ cup extra virgin olive oil

2 tablespoons filtered water

2 tablespoons rice wine vinegar

2½ teaspoons ume plum vinegar

2 tablespoons toasted sesame oil

2 tablespoons chopped fresh cilantro

½ shallot, minced (2 tablespoons)

1 tablespoon micro-grated peeled ginger

1 tablespoon nutritional yeast

¼ teaspoon black pepper

1. Combine all ingredients in a high-speed blender and blend well until smooth and creamy. Store, refrigerated, in a glass jar for up to 1 week.

Clean Ketchup

Makes: 1 cup

Prep Time: 5 minutes

1 (6-ounce) can tomato paste

2 tablespoons gluten-free tamari

1 tablespoon apple cider vinegar

2 teaspoons raw honey (optional)

½ teaspoon ground allspice

¼ teaspoon chipotle chili powder

½ teaspoon sea salt

Ketchup is a staple in every American household, but did you know it's usually packed with sugar and artificial ingredients? I created this version as a flavorful, healthy alternative so you can elevate your favorite dishes and throw the other stuff away. I especially love serving it with my Crispy Carrot Fries (page 155).

1. Scoop out the tomato paste and place it in a small bowl. Add the remaining ingredients and stir well to combine. Store in an airtight container in the fridge for up to 1 week.

Coconut Chutney

CONTRIBUTED BY MARK BITTMAN

Makes: 1 cup

Prep Time: 10 minutes

½ cup unsweetened
shredded coconut

1 (1-inch) piece fresh ginger,
peeled and chopped; or
1 teaspoon ground ginger

1 hot fresh green or red chile;
or red chili flakes to taste

½ bunch fresh cilantro,
leaves only

¼ teaspoon ground cumin

2 tablespoons fresh lime juice

Salt to taste

This recipe comes from my friend Mark Bittman, a food journalist, and was featured in his amazing book *How to Cook Everything Vegetarian.* It's a refreshing way to spice up a variety of dishes, especially those that are Indian-inspired. Mark says if you don't have coconut on hand, or don't prefer it, swap in chopped carrots or beets for an equally delicious condiment.

1. Combine the coconut, ginger, chile, cilantro, and cumin in a food processor or blender and pulse until finely ground.

2. Add the lime juice and a pinch of salt and pulse again, until nearly but not quite smooth. Taste and adjust the seasoning as needed. Serve at room temperature. Best enjoyed the same day.

Dairy-Free Queso

Makes: 2 cups

Prep Time: 5 minutes,
plus 4 hours soaking

Cook Time: 10 minutes

¾ cup plus 2 tablespoons
raw sunflower seeds

2 tablespoons avocado oil

1 medium white onion, finely
chopped (about 2 cups)

2 tablespoons chopped fresh
thyme

1 teaspoon sea salt, plus
more for seasoning

½ cup filtered water

⅓ cup nutritional yeast

1 tablespoon brown rice miso

1 teaspoon Dijon mustard

¼ teaspoon smoked paprika

¼ teaspoon onion powder

¼ teaspoon freshly ground
black pepper, plus more for
seasoning

This cheesy sauce will become a new family favorite. It's especially good slathered on broccoli, tossed with steamed or roasted vegetables, or used as a dip for roasted sweet potato rounds. Soaked and blended sunflower seeds make a rich, creamy base to carry the aromatic flavors of onion and thyme. Nutritional yeast is a useful ingredient for mimicking the taste of cheese while providing an impressive array of B vitamins.

1. Soak the sunflower seeds in filtered water for 4 hours. Rinse well and drain.

2. Heat the avocado oil in a large skillet over medium heat until shimmering. Add the onion and cook for 5 minutes. Add the thyme and salt and cook for another 5 minutes, until the onions are fragrant and translucent.

3. Transfer the onion mixture to a high-speed blender and add the sunflower seeds, water, nutritional yeast, miso, mustard, smoked paprika, onion powder, and black pepper. Blend until smooth and creamy, then season with more salt and pepper to taste. Store leftovers in a glass container in the fridge for up to 5 days.

Easy Homemade Teriyaki Sauce

Makes: 1 cup

Prep Time: 5 minutes
Cook Time: 12 minutes

2 teaspoons avocado oil

4 cloves garlic, micro-grated

1 tablespoon micro-grated peeled fresh ginger

1 pinch chili flakes

⅔ cup gluten-free tamari or coconut aminos

¼ cup plus 2 tablespoons filtered water

¼ cup mirin

¼ cup rice wine vinegar

Store-bought teriyaki sauce is filled with sugar—and usually gluten, too. This homemade sauce is a delicious alternative, super simple to make and perfect for a quick stir-fry. It's also a great dressing for cabbage or broccoli salad.

1. Heat the avocado oil in a small saucepan over low heat. Add the garlic, ginger, and chili flakes and gently sauté for 2 minutes.

2. Add the tamari and water and bring to a simmer. Simmer on low for 8 minutes. Add the mirin and vinegar and simmer for 2 minutes longer.

3. Strain the sauce through a fine-mesh sieve to remove solids. Store in a glass jar in the fridge for up to 1 week.

Everything Vinaigrette

Makes: 1 cup

Prep Time: 10 minutes

½ cup raw walnuts

¾ cup extra virgin olive oil

1 teaspoon toasted sesame oil

¼ cup balsamic vinegar

1 tablespoon Dijon mustard

1 clove garlic, peeled

½ teaspoon sea salt

¼ teaspoon freshly ground black pepper

This vinaigrette works with any salad or vegetable dish, which is good news because you'll honestly want to put it on everything! It's also great drizzled over steak or chicken. Store-bought dressings are full of inflammatory oils, preservatives, hidden sugar, and often gluten. But this one is rich in healthy omega-3 and monounsaturated fats and is incredibly flavorful thanks to the unique addition of toasted walnuts.

1. In a small pan, toast the walnuts for 4 minutes over medium heat, until golden and fragrant. Remove from the heat and set aside to cool.

2. Combine the toasted walnuts, olive oil, sesame oil, vinegar, mustard, garlic, salt, and pepper in a food processor. Purée until creamy but not completely smooth; I like to keep a little texture from the walnuts. Store in a glass jar in the fridge for up to 1 week.

Greek Spice Rub

Makes: 1 cup

Prep Time: 5 minutes

2 tablespoons garlic powder

2 tablespoons dried oregano

2½ tablespoons onion powder

1½ tablespoons dried basil

1½ tablespoons dried dill

1½ tablespoons dried parsley

1 tablespoon dried rosemary

1 tablespoon dried thyme

1½ teaspoons dried lemon zest

1½ teaspoons grated nutmeg

½ teaspoon ground cinnamon

1 tablespoon plus 1 teaspoon
sea salt

1 tablespoon freshly ground
black pepper

This simple spice blend embraces the traditional flavors of Greek fare, some of the healthiest food on the planet. It's perfect sprinkled over chicken thighs or tossed with roasted mushrooms, zucchini, and onions.

1. Mix all ingredients together in a small bowl and store in an airtight container for up to 1 year.

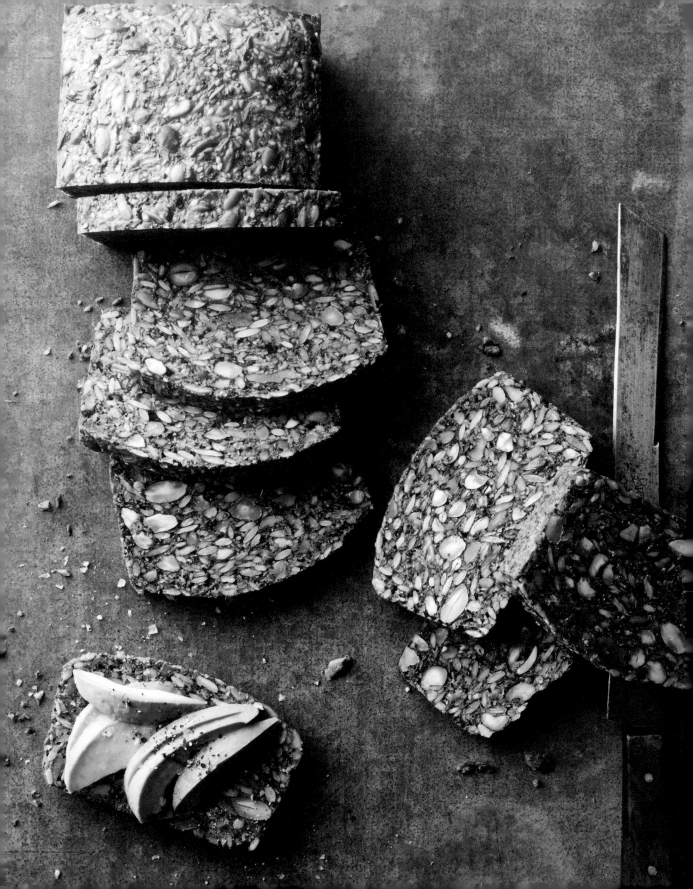

Flourless Protein Power Bread

Serves: 8

Prep Time: 5 minutes
Cook Time: 50 to
60 minutes

⅓ cup plus 1 tablespoon
avocado oil

⅔ cup raw almonds

⅔ cup raw hazelnuts

⅔ cup raw walnuts

⅓ cup raw pistachios

⅔ cup raw sunflower seeds

⅔ cup raw pumpkin seeds

¼ cup raw sesame seeds

¼ cup hemp seeds

¼ cup chia seeds

½ cup whole flaxseeds

2 tablespoons cumin seeds
(optional)

6 large pasture-raised eggs

½ teaspoon apple cider vinegar

1½ teaspoons sea salt

You won't believe how delicious and easy this bread is. Made from nourishing nuts, seeds, and eggs, it's got plenty of healthy fats and protein. Try it warm with some mashed avocado or a slather of ghee or coconut butter. I like to make two loaves at a time so I always have some in the freezer: Wrap slices in parchment paper and tinfoil, place in a sealed container, and freeze for up to 2 months. Simply unwrap and toast for a few minutes when you're ready to enjoy!

1. Preheat the oven to 350°F. Use 1 tablespoon of the avocado oil to grease an 8½ x 4½-inch loaf pan.

2. In a food processor, combine the almonds, hazelnuts, walnuts, and pistachios. Pulse 7 times until chunky; be careful not to overprocess.

3. In a bowl, mix the sunflower seeds, pumpkin seeds, sesame seeds, hemp seeds, chia seeds, flaxseeds, and cumin seeds (if using). Add the processed nut mixture and stir to combine.

4. In a separate bowl, beat the remaining ⅓ cup avocado oil with the eggs, vinegar, and salt. Add the nut and seed mixture and mix well.

5. Pour the batter into the greased loaf pan. Bake for 50 to 60 minutes, until a toothpick inserted in the middle comes out clean. Allow the bread to cool before slicing.

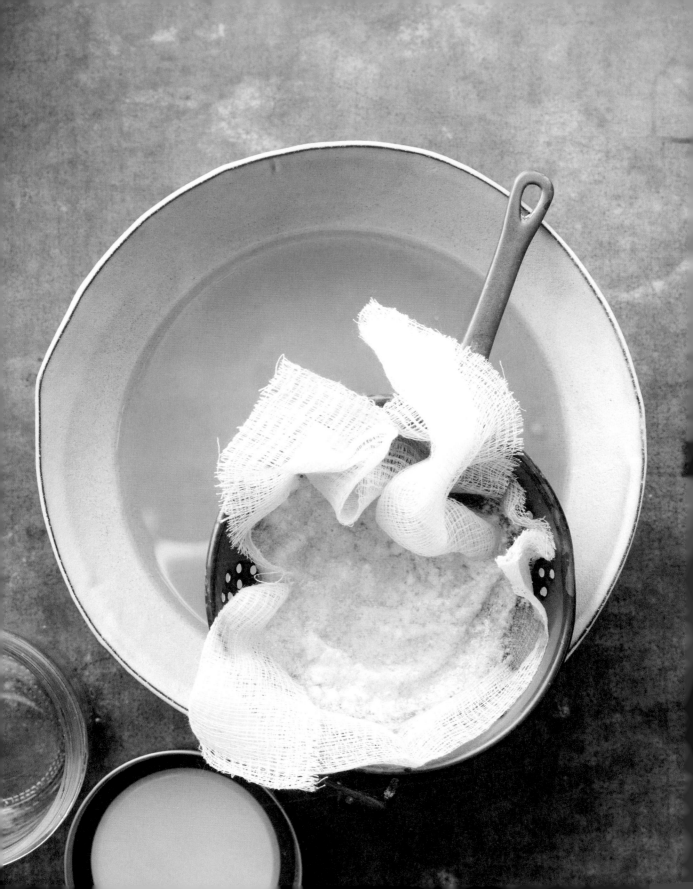

Grass-Fed Ghee

Makes: 2 cups

Prep Time: 2 minutes
Cook Time: 30 minutes

1 pound unsalted butter,
cut into cubes

Ghee is highly clarified butter, meaning the milk solids have been removed from the fat. This leaves it with little to no lactose, so it is often better tolerated by those who are sensitive. Ghee is also a helpful kitchen staple to have on hand because it adds loads of flavor to any dish, and its stable fats make it an excellent choice for high-heat cooking. Make sure to look for grass-fed butter to get the most nutrition out of your homemade ghee!

1. In a small saucepan, warm the butter over medium heat until completely melted and beginning to simmer. Reduce the heat to low and cook, without stirring, until the foam settles to the bottom of the pan, about 20 minutes.

2. Line a fine-mesh sieve with cheesecloth and set over a bowl. Strain the ghee through the sieve, then transfer to a glass jar and seal tightly. Store at room temperature for up to 30 days, or in the refrigerator for up to 6 months.

Makes: 1½ cups

Prep Time: 10 minutes

½ cup fresh flat-leaf parsley leaves, chopped

½ cup fresh cilantro leaves, chopped

½ cup lemon juice

½ cup extra virgin olive oil

1 small avocado, pitted and peeled

2 tablespoons chopped green onion

2 teaspoons Dijon mustard

3 cloves garlic, micro-grated

¾ teaspoon sea salt

Pinch of black pepper

Green Goodness Dressing

The name of this dressing says it all—it's so good! And it's easy to make. A variety of green herbs provide plenty of phytonutrients, and when blended with rich avocado and olive oil, they create a beautiful, bright, creamy dressing that you'll want to have in the fridge at all times.

1. Combine all ingredients in a blender and purée until smooth. Pour into a glass jar and store in the fridge for up to 1 week.

Out-of-This-World Alfredo

Makes: 2½ cups

Prep Time: 5 minutes,
plus 4 hours soaking

Cook Time: 25 minutes

2 tablespoons avocado oil

3 cups finely diced button
mushrooms

½ red onion, diced

4 cloves garlic, chopped

1 cup raw cashews, soaked
4 hours or overnight,
drained and rinsed

1 cup filtered water

1 teaspoon grated lemon zest

1 tablespoon lemon juice

1¼ teaspoons sea salt

¼ teaspoon freshly ground
black pepper

You won't miss dairy one bit when you taste this creamy cashew-based sauce. Mushrooms and garlic create intense flavor while also contributing tons of immune-boosting phytonutrients. Toss with your favorite veggie noodles or serve with roasted broccoli.

1. Heat 1 tablespoon of the avocado oil in a large skillet over low-medium heat until shimmering. Add the mushrooms and sauté until soft, 8 to 10 minutes. Remove the mushrooms from the pan and set aside.

2. Add the remaining 1 tablespoon avocado oil to the pan, then add the onion and cook down over medium-low heat for 8 minutes. Add the garlic and cashews and sauté for 2 minutes.

3. In a blender, combine ⅓ cup of the cooked mushrooms, the sautéed cashew mix, water, lemon zest and juice, salt, and pepper and purée until smooth.

4. Pour the sauce back into the pan, add the remaining cooked mushrooms, and stir well over medium heat for several minutes, until combined and warm. Store cooled leftovers in a glass jar in the fridge for up to 1 week.

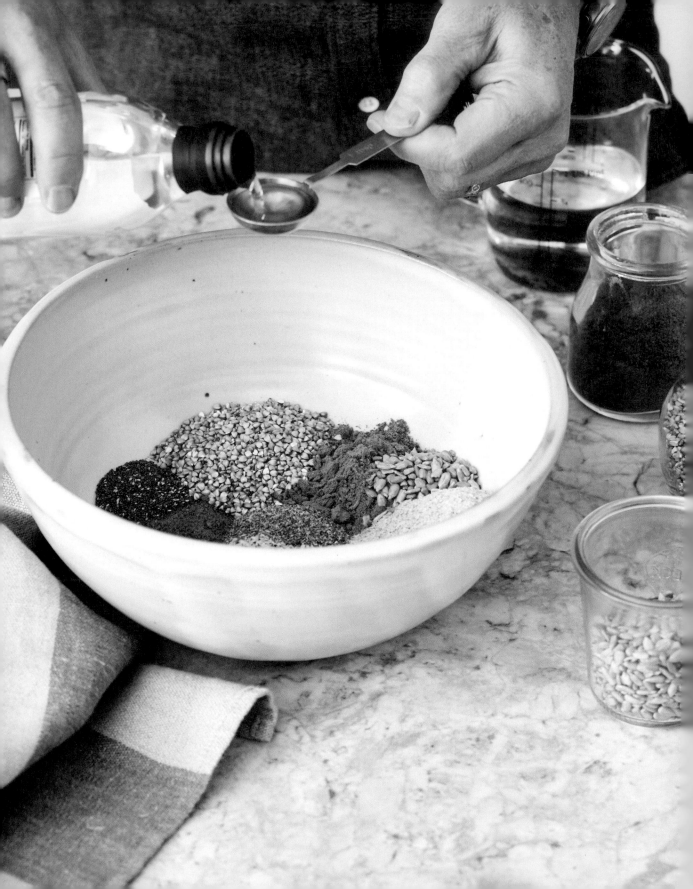

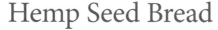

Hemp Seed Bread

CONTRIBUTED BY CAM SIMS

This recipe is from my friend Cam Sims of New Zealand, the hemp-based chef and founder of Plant Culture, a company devoted to producing conscious hemp seed products. Cam's bread is packed full of protein, fiber, minerals, and omega-3 fats. It is whole-food, gluten-free, Paleo, and self-activating too. It is also great for the gut. The combination of hemp, flax, chia, buckwheat, and psyllium husk provides prebiotic fiber, which helps optimize your microbiome. Pre-slice it, freeze it. Toast it. Love it.

Serves: 8

Prep Time: 10 minutes, plus 2 hours seed activating, if desired

Cook Time: 50 to 60 minutes

¾ cup hemp seeds

⅓ cup hemp protein

⅓ cup raw sunflower seeds

½ cup ground flaxseed

¾ cup raw buckwheat groats

2 tablespoons chia seeds

¼ cup psyllium seed husks; or 3 tablespoons psyllium husk powder

3 tablespoons coconut sugar

1 teaspoon fine grain sea salt; or 1½ teaspoons coarse salt

3 tablespoons hemp seed oil or coconut oil, melted

1½ cups filtered water

VARIATIONS

Rosemary: Add 2 tablespoons dried rosemary or minced fresh rosemary with the hemp seeds in the first step.

Chocolate: Add ½ cup pitted, chopped dates, ¾ cup cocoa powder, and ½ cup filtered water with the hemp seeds in the first step.

1. Combine the hemp seeds, hemp protein, sunflower seeds, flaxseed, buckwheat groats, chia seeds, psyllium, coconut sugar, and sea salt in a large bowl and mix well. In a medium bowl, mix the hemp seed oil and water together, then quickly add to the dry ingredients. Mix wet and dry ingredients thoroughly until thick and well combined.

2. Line an 8½ x 4½-inch loaf pan with parchment paper, add the seed mixture, and smooth the top with the back of a wet spoon. If you want to activate the seeds, let the container sit on the counter for at least 2 hours; or, if you have time, allow it to rest overnight, covered, at room temperature. Otherwise, move on to baking.

3. When ready to bake, preheat the oven to 355°F.

4. Bake the loaf on the oven's middle rack for 20 minutes. Remove the bread from the pan and place upside down directly on the middle rack. Bake for 30 to 40 minutes longer. The bread is ready when tapping it with your knuckle produces a hollow sound.

5. Let cool completely before slicing. Store the bread in a sealed container for up to 5 days. The best way to store this bread is by pre-slicing it all and freezing in an airtight container for up to 6 months. Defrost slices using the toaster or oven.

Immune-Boosting Bone Broth

Makes: 8 cups

Prep Time: 20 minutes
Cook Time: 40 minutes,
plus 8 to 24 hours in
the slow cooker or on the
stovetop

4 pounds grass-fed beef
marrow bones, cut in half
by a butcher

2 pounds meaty bones from
grass-fed beef, such as short
ribs, shank, or oxtail

1 large carrot, unpeeled,
roughly chopped

1 leek, ends trimmed,
roughly chopped

2 yellow onions with skin,
quartered

1 parsnip, peeled and
roughly chopped

1 celery root, peeled and
quartered

1 head garlic with peel,
halved crosswise

15 cups filtered water,
plus more if necessary

½ cup apple cider vinegar

2 celery stalks, roughly
chopped

2 fennel bulbs, quartered

2 star anise

2 bay leaves

1 tablespoon sea salt

2 tablespoons whole
black peppercorns

Bone broth is an ultra-healing food that is traditional in many cultures. Stewing bones for long periods of time with vinegar and herbs draws out protein, collagen, and minerals that benefit your skin, joints, gut, detox processes, and more. Use the broth as a base for soups and stews, drink some as a meal, or simply sip throughout the day for an extra nutritional boost.

1. Preheat the oven to 450°F.

2. Combine the beef bones, carrot, leek, onions, parsnip, celery root, and garlic in a roasting pan and roast for 20 minutes. Toss the contents of the pan, then continue to roast another 20 minutes, until caramelized.

3. In a large slow cooker, combine the water, vinegar, celery, fennel, star anise, bay leaves, salt, and peppercorns. Scrape the roasted bones and vegetables into the pot along with any juices. (Alternatively, combine everything in a large pot on the stovetop.)

4. Cover the slow cooker or pot and cook on low for at least 8 hours or up to 24 hours. Skim and discard the foam and peels that rise to the top as the broth cooks. (As always, take extra care if leaving the stove on for an extended period of time.) The longer you cook, the more collagen and protein you'll pull from the bones.

5. When the broth is ready, let cool to room temperature, then strain through a fine-mesh sieve. Refrigerate overnight. The broth should be gelatinous when chilled. Remove solidified fat from the top.

6. Reheat when ready to enjoy. Leftovers can be stored for 3 to 4 days in the fridge, or several months in the freezer. You can even freeze broth in ice cube trays for handy cubes that make a flavorful addition to soups and sauces.

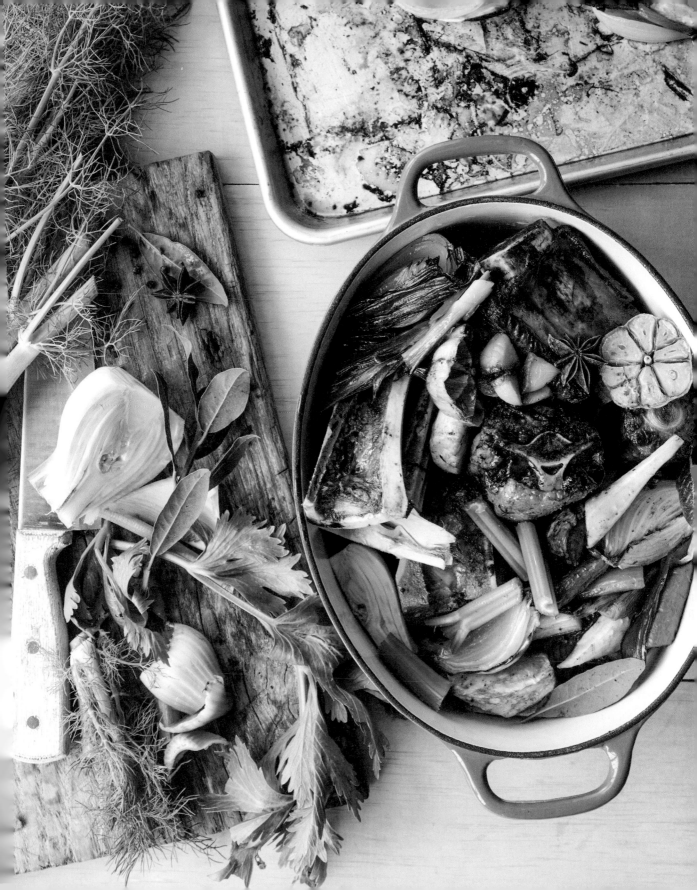

Pumpkin Cilantro Pesto

Makes: 1½ cups

Prep Time: 10 minutes
Cook Time: 5 minutes

1 cup pepitas, toasted

2 cups loosely packed
fresh cilantro, chopped

2 cloves garlic, pressed

1½ teaspoons chopped
seeded jalapeño

⅓ cup extra virgin olive oil

2 tablespoons lemon juice

2 teaspoons gluten-free
tamari or coconut aminos

1 tablespoon nutritional yeast

½ teaspoon sea salt

This pesto is full of nutrients and beneficial phytocompounds: Pepitas (green pumpkin seeds) are bursting with minerals such as magnesium, manganese, phosphorus, and iron; cilantro helps the body detoxify heavy metals. With spicy jalapeño, pungent garlic, and tart lemon juice, this unique take on pesto is a rich and flavorful dip for fresh-cut vegetables, like carrots or cucumbers, plus it's a breeze to make.

1. Heat a large sauté pan over medium-high heat. Add the pepitas and stir frequently until fragrant and toasted, about 5 minutes. Remove from the heat and set aside.

2. Combine the toasted pepitas and all the remaining ingredients in a high-speed blender or food processor and purée until a chunky dip is created. You may need to add 1 to 2 tablespoons water to help it blend. Store leftovers in a glass container for up to 5 days.

Savory Seed Crackers

Makes: About 60
(2-inch) crackers

Prep Time: 15 minutes
plus cooling
Cook Time: 1 hour
20 minutes

1 cup brown basmati rice

1 cup raw buckwheat groats

4 cups filtered water

½ cup raw sunflower seeds

¼ cup whole brown flaxseeds

¼ cup chia seeds

1 tablespoon Italian seasoning

1 teaspoon garlic powder

2 tablespoons miso paste

I love having these crispy crackers on hand for a quick snack. They've got omega-3 fats, fiber, and plant-based protein, all wrapped up in a satisfying, crunchy cracker. One of my favorite ways to serve them is with my spicy Blushing Beet Dip (page 149) and chopped veggies.

1. In a medium saucepan, bring the rice, buckwheat, and water to a boil. Cover, reduce the heat to low, and cook for 20 minutes. Remove from the heat and let stand for 10 minutes; the water should be completely absorbed. Spread the mixture out on a baking sheet, and let cool completely.

2. Preheat the oven to 350°F.

3. Once cooled, transfer the rice and buckwheat mixture to a food processor and process until a chunky dough is formed. Add the sunflower seeds, flaxseeds, chia seeds, Italian seasoning, garlic powder, and miso and continue to process until everything is thoroughly combined.

4. Transfer half of the dough to a sheet of parchment paper. Place another sheet of parchment or plastic wrap on top. Using a rolling pin, roll the dough to a ¼-inch-thick, 10 x 12-inch rectangle. Remove the top layer of parchment or plastic. Score the dough into 2-inch squares. Transfer the dough and the bottom layer of parchment to a baking sheet. Repeat with the other half of dough.

5. Bake until the tops are beginning to brown and feel dry to the touch, about 25 minutes. Flip the crackers, rotate the baking sheets between the oven racks, and continue to bake for another 25 to 30 minutes, until the crackers are firm when pressed. Remove from the oven and cool on a rack. The crackers will continue to crisp as they cool. Once completely cooled, separate the crackers where scored and store in an airtight container for up to 2 weeks.

Smoky Chipotle Ranch Dressing

CONTRIBUTED BY MARK SISSON

Makes: 1¾ cups

Prep Time: 5 minutes

1 cup Primal Kitchen Avocado Mayo

½ cup full-fat unsweetened coconut milk

Juice of 2 lemons

2 teaspoons onion powder

1 tablespoon garlic powder

2 teaspoons chipotle powder

½ teaspoon sea salt

1 tablespoon plus 2 teaspoons tightly packed minced fresh parsley

2 tablespoons fresh chives, minced

There's nothing quite like a creamy dressing to make veggies pop. This smoky ranch from my friend Mark Sisson, founder of Primal Kitchen, is amazing over salads and roasted veggies, and even when used as a dip. The chipotle gives it a subtle kick and the herbs lend an extra layer of fresh flavor, while also adding beneficial phytonutrients.

1. Combine the avocado mayo, coconut milk, lemon juice, onion powder, garlic powder, chipotle powder, and salt in a blender and blend until smooth.

2. Stir in the parsley and chives and pour the dressing into a glass jar. Store in the fridge for up to 1 week.

Tangy Tomato Basil Sauce

Makes: 5 cups

Prep Time: 5 minutes, plus 30 minutes resting

Cook Time: 1 hour 15 minutes

2 medium red bell peppers

2 tablespoons avocado oil

1 medium red onion, finely chopped

2 tablespoons pressed garlic

¾ cup sundried tomatoes, finely minced

⅓ cup capers, minced

1 teaspoon sea salt

1 cup fresh basil leaves, finely chopped

¼ cup tomato paste

1 (28-ounce) can diced tomatoes

1 teaspoon balsamic vinegar

Chili flakes (optional)

Tomato sauce is a must-have kitchen staple, but did you know most store-bought pasta sauces contain lots of added sugar and preservatives? Keep a batch of this homemade sauce on hand at all times for a quick weeknight meal. Toss with your favorite veggie noodles—perhaps with ground beef or turkey. It's also perfect over roasted cauliflower.

1. Preheat the oven to 450°F. Line a baking sheet with parchment. Cut the peppers in half, then remove the seeds and core. Lay flat, skin side down, on the lined baking sheet. Roast for 45 minutes, or until the skins are slightly blackened. Transfer the roasted peppers to a bowl, cover, and let sit for 30 minutes. Pull off the black skin and chop the peppers into small pieces.

2. Heat the avocado oil in a medium sauté pan over medium heat until shimmering. Add the onion and sauté for 10 minutes, until translucent. Add the garlic, sundried tomatoes, capers, and salt and cook for another 5 minutes, until fragrant and the garlic is lightly browned. Add the roasted peppers, basil, and tomato paste and stir for 2 minutes. Add the diced tomatoes and let the mixture simmer for 15 minutes, stirring occasionally.

3. Remove from the heat and stir in the balsamic vinegar. Sprinkle with chili flakes if desired. Store leftovers in a glass jar in the fridge for up to 1 week.

Turmeric Oil

CONTRIBUTED BY CHEF DAVID BOULEY

Makes: 2⅓ cups

Prep Time: 5 minutes
plus 2 hours infusing

Cook Time: 30 minutes

2⅓ cups avocado oil

2 tablespoons plus
½ teaspoon ground turmeric

4 black peppercorns

This delicious antioxidant-rich oil comes from my very talented friend, Chef David Bouley. Turmeric oil is a great staple to have on hand for drizzling over anything—from veggies to poultry to fish—and it's a nourishing way to add tons of flavor and anti-inflammatory properties to a dish.

1. Mix the oil and turmeric in a small saucepan and cook over very low heat, keeping the temperature at 150°F, for 30 minutes. Add the peppercorns, turn off the heat, and cover with a lid. Let the oil infuse for 2 hours while cooling. Store in a glass jar in a dark cabinet for up to 1 month.

Zesty Mexican Seasoning

Makes: 1 cup

Prep Time: 5 minutes

¼ cup plus 1 tablespoon chili powder

2½ tablespoons garlic powder

2 tablespoons dried oregano

2 tablespoons ground cumin

2 tablespoons onion powder

1 tablespoon paprika

1½ teaspoons smoked paprika

1 teaspoon chili flakes

1 tablespoon sea salt

2 teaspoons black pepper

Having delicious spice blends on hand makes healthy home cooking a breeze. I love using this simple seasoning on everything from chicken and steak to cauliflower and zucchini. Or use it for lettuce wraps, Southwestern veggie bowls, or even a unique spin on scrambled eggs.

1. Mix all the ingredients in a small bowl; store in an airtight container for up to 1 year.

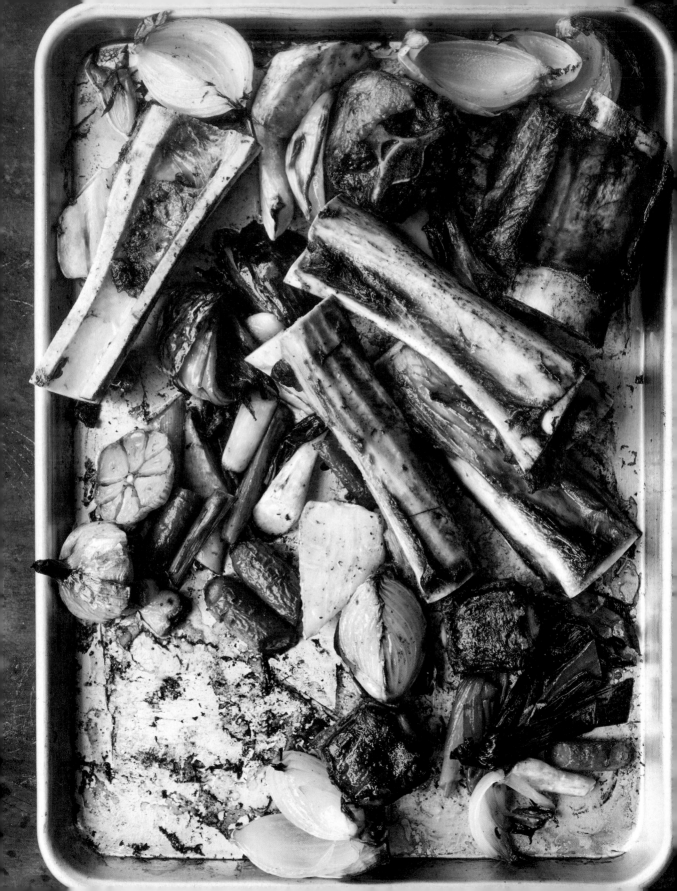

ACKNOWLEDGMENTS

Writing this cookbook was a way for me to encourage others to participate in a revolutionary act—cooking—and to show just how delicious and fun making meals from real, wholesome food can be. Cooking has always been a way for me to show love to others, and it's become a cornerstone of how I teach my patients to love themselves.

After writing my last book, *Food: What the Heck Should I Eat?*, I wanted to continue the conversation about ending nutritional confusion once and for all—this time by providing the step-by-step processes for making nutritious homemade meals. It is my hope that the amazing recipes in this book will propel you to change your own life for the better.

None of this would be possible without the support of you, my community, the people who share my belief in the medicinal power of food. We are working together to change the course of public health and the food system as we know it. Thank you for joining me in this cause.

Many thanks to Chef Mikaela Reuben and Chef Frank Giglio for helping me create these delectable meals; I greatly appreciate your shared passion for real food and the time and skill you both devoted to this project. I also want to thank photographer Nicole Franzen, food stylist Vivian Lui, and prop stylist Joni Noe for bringing these recipes to life with your beautiful photos.

I'm so grateful to all my friends who contributed recipes: Cam Sims, Chef David Bouley, Chef José Andrés, Chef Marco Canora, Danielle Walker, Dave Asprey, Dr. David and Mrs. Leize Perlmutter, Dr. Deanna Minich, Dr. Drew Ramsey, Dr. Mehmet Oz, Dr. Terry Wahls, Dr. Rupy Aujla, Gisele Bündchen and Tom Brady, Gwyneth Paltrow, Hugh Jackman, Kris Carr, Mark Bittman, and Mark Sisson; thank you for sharing your delicious creations.

And, of course, I need to thank my team. Kaya Purohit, thank you for helping me bring all my projects to fruition and for being a sounding board for the cookbook team. Ronit Menashe, you played an essential role in organizing the team and carrying out my vision. Thank you Ayelet Menashe for sharing your culinary expertise in recipe development and your help with the planning process. Ailsa Cowell, thank you for sharing your passion for real food and nutrition in each page of this book and for managing the many moving parts of this project. To my assistant Meredith Jones, thank you for keeping my life organized and always moving in the right direction. And I can't forget my business partner, Dhru Purohit—thank you for being such a positive force behind our team and for providing the support to make this all happen! I'd also like to thank the rest of the Hyman Digital team for helping me share the power of real food with others.

Thank you to my team at Little, Brown for making this all possible, especially my editor Tracy Behar, for still believing in my message after twenty years. And to my agent Richard Pine, who has also guided my work for the past two decades, thank you for supporting my dreams.

And last but never least, my wife, Mia. Thank you for being my rock and encouraging me in everything I do; I'm forever grateful.

RESOURCES

Clean Seafood

Natural Resources Defense Council (nrdc.org/stores/smart-seafood-buying-guide): An easy-to-use guide on how to buy fish that is good for you and the environment.

Marine Stewardship Council (msc.org): Nonprofit covering traceable, sustainable seafood while focusing on keeping the oceans full and abundant.

Clean Fish (cleanfish.com): Resource for farmed fish that have zero antibiotics and hormones, low mercury content, and high levels of omega-3s. This is essential if you plan to eat farmed fish.

EWG's *Consumer Guide to Seafood* (ewg.org/research/ewgs-good-seafood-guide): A wonderful resource for determining what kinds of seafoods are safest to eat and which should be avoided.

Fair Trade and Rainforest Alliance Certified

Fair Trade Federation (fairtradefederation.org): Information on the Fair Trade movement and verified Fair Trade wholesalers.

World Fair Trade Organization (wfto.com): A resource for reporting Fair Trade non-compliance, finding trustworthy suppliers, and getting involved in the movement.

Equal Exchange (equalexchange.coop/about): An importer and distributer for Fair Trade worker cooperatives that benefit farmers and offer a variety of socially responsible products.

Fair Trade International (fairtrade.net): Information on Fair Trade labeling requirements and which products you can trust.

Rainforest Alliance (rainforest-alliance.org): A great resource for understanding the links between environmental degradation, agriculture, and social well-being.

Gluten-Free

Celiac.com: Comprehensive website on all things celiac, including a list of gluten's many names and the foods it can hide in.

Grass-Fed and Pasture-Raised Foods

American Grassfed Association (americangrassfed.org/producer-profiles): Directory of approved producers of grass-fed meat by state.

Kiss the Ground (kisstheground.com): Book and movie highlighting the positive effects of regenerative agriculture on the climate, soil, water, and even drought and flood patterns, as well as the benefits of raising animals on a wholesome diet and with the ability to move freely.

Eatwild (eatwild.com/products): Directory of pasture-based farms throughout the country, including poultry, eggs, and grass-fed meat or dairy.

Local Harvest (localharvest.org): An amazing resource for all things local, including grass-fed beef, poultry, eggs, and produce.

EWG's *Meat Eater's Guide to Climate Change and Health* (ewg.org/meateatersguide/eat -smart): An extensive guide to meat-related labeling, certification, and best practices for being a conscious meat eater.

CAFO (cafothebook.org): Information about the practices of industrial animal agriculture, also known as concentrated animal feeding operations, and the risks it presents to public health and the environment, as well as the harm and mistreatment it brings upon the animals raised for our food.

Eat Well Guide (eatwellguide.org): Resources for finding sustainably raised poultry and eggs at a wide variety of locations, from supermarkets to websites.

Butcher Box (butcherbox.com/drhyman-fans): A great resource for buying grass-fed, pasture-raised, and organic animal products online. Receive $10 off your first order and free shipping.

Local

National Farmers Market Directory (ams.usda.gov/local-food-directories/farmersmarkets): Directory of markets in many areas, as well as what they offer, business hours, accepted forms of payment, and more.

Local Harvest (localharvest.org/csa): A great resource for discovering CSA programs near you.

Imperfect Produce (imperfectproduce.com): Company that works with local farmers to deliver perfectly edible "ugly" produce that can't be sold at supermarkets to your front door at a deeply discounted rate. Currently serving the Bay Area, Los Angeles, Seattle, Portland, and Chicago, with more regions coming soon.

Hungry Harvest (hungryharvest.net): A wonderful resource for finding discounted surplus produce from CSA programs. Plus, for every box you buy, one is donated to a family in need.

Non-GMO

EWG's *Shoppers Guide to Avoiding GMOs* (ewg.org/research/shoppers-guide-to-avoiding -gmos): Safety information regarding GMOs and additional tips on how to avoid them.

Non-GMO Project (nongmoproject.org): A comprehensive resource with up-to-date information on non-GMO labeling initiatives and safe products.

Organic

EWG's Dirty Dozen and Clean Fifteen (ewg.org): Printable versions of the Dirty Dozen and Clean Fifteen lists to use the next time you're navigating the produce section.

Organic Consumers Association (organicconsumers.org): Up-to-date information on organic policy initiatives, social and environmental issues, product information, and more on all things organic.

USDA National Organic Program (NOP) (ams.usda.gov/rules-regulations/organic): Updates on food labeling; currently in the process of developing labeling standards.

Healthy Eating and Our Food System

Nina Teicholz (thebigfatsurprise.com): An investigative journalist who writes about food misconceptions. Her work led Congress to mandate a review of the food guidelines by the National Academy of Sciences and the influences the food industry had on these guidelines.

Dariush Mozaffarian (wbur.org/commonhealth/2018/04/03/tufts-nutritionist-eating -healthy): Interview with the dean of the Friedman School of Nutrition Science and Policy at Tufts University on dietary guidelines, food policy, and public health.

For more on me (drhyman.com): Many useful resources including podcasts, articles, videos, and recipes, and check out my last book, *Food: What the Heck Should I Eat?*, which addresses the influence of food industry lobbying on our public health policy, that lobby misleading people into making bad food choices, and the science behind different diets.

Healthy Online Shopping

Dry Farm Wines (dryfarmwines.com): A wine club focused on biodynamic, additive-free, sugar-free, low-alcohol wines that are lab tested for purity. Create your own case of 6 to 12 bottles and have it delivered right to your home with complimentary shipping.

Thrive Market (thrivemarket.com): Membership-based online community that delivers high-quality healthy food and natural products to your doorstep—at wholesale prices. Savings can be anywhere from 25 to 50 percent off average retail prices for your favorite items. And for every membership purchased, Thrive donates one to a low-income family, teacher, veteran, or student to help make healthy living easy and affordable for everyone.

Our Contributors

Chef José Andrés: thinkfoodgroup.com

Dave Asprey: bulletproof.com

Dr. Rupy Aujla: thedoctorskitchen.com

Mark Bittman: markbittman.com

Chef David Bouley: davidbouley.com

Gisele Bündchen and Tom Brady: instagram.com/gisele and instagram.com/tombrady

Chef Marco Canora: restauranthearth.com /team-member/executive-chef

Kris Carr: kriscarr.com

Hugh Jackman: instagram.com /thehughjackman

Dr. Deanna Minich: deannaminich.com

Dr. Mehmet Oz: doctoroz.com

Gwyneth Paltrow: goop.com

Dr. David Perlmutter and Leize Perlmutter: drperlmutter.com

Dr. Drew Ramsey: drewramseymd.com

Cam Sims: plantculture.nz

Mark Sisson: primalkitchen.com/pages /about

Dr. Terry Wahls: terrywahls.com

Danielle Walker: againstallgrain.com

NOTES

Learning How to Eat

1. Nestle M. Food marketing and childhood obesity—a matter of policy. *N Engl J Med.* 2006 Jun 15;354(24):2517–29.

2. Freeman A. Fast food: Oppression through poor nutrition, 95 *Calif. L. Rev.* 2221 (2007).

3. Kessler DA. Toward more comprehensive food labeling. *N Engl J Med.* 2014 Jul 17;371(3):193–95.

4. Union of Concerned Scientists. Hidden cost of industrial agriculture. https://www.ucsusa.org/food_and_agriculture/our-failing-food-system/industrial-agriculture/hidden-costs-of-industrial.html#.W2kMGthKjOQ. Accessed September 1, 2018.

5. *The Guardian.* Prison study could show better diet reduces violence. https://www.theguardian.com/society/2008/jan/29/prisonsandprobation.foodanddrink. January 29, 2008.

6. Craig WJ. Health effects of vegan diets. *Am J Clinical Nutr.* 2009 May;89(5):1627S–1633S, https://doi.org/10.3945/ajcn.2009.26736N.

7. Klonoff DC. The beneficial effects of a Paleolithic Diet on type 2 diabetes and other risk factors for cardiovascular disease. *J Diabetes Sci Technol.* 2009 Nov;3(6):1229–32, doi:10.1177/193229680900300601.

8. Fasano A, Sapone A, Zevallos V, Schuppan D. Nonceliac gluten sensitivity. *Gastroenterology.* 2015 May;128(6):1195–1204.

9. Ludwig DS, Willett WC. Three daily servings of reduced-fat milk: An evidence-based recommendation: *JAMA Pediatr.* 2013;167(9):788–89.

10. Ebbeling CB, Swain JF, Feldman HA, et al. Effects of dietary composition on energy expenditure during weight-loss maintenance. *JAMA.* 2012 Jun 27;307(24):2627–34.

11. Avena NM, Rada P, Hoebel BG. Evidence for sugar addiction: Behavioral and neurochemical effects of intermittent, excessive sugar intake. *Neurosci Biobehav Rev.* 2008; 32(1):20–39. doi:10.1016/j.neubiorev.2007.04.019

12. Whalen KA, Judd S, McCullough ML, Flanders WD, Hartman TJ, Bostick RM. Paleolithic and Mediterranean diet pattern scores are inversely associated with all-cause and cause-specific mortality in adults. *J Nutr.* 2017 Feb 8.

13. US Department of Health and Human Services; US Department of Agriculture. Scientific Report of the 2015 Dietary Guidelines Advisory Committee. Washington, DC; February 2015.

14. Freed DLJ. Do dietary lectins cause disease? *BMJ.* 1999 Apr 17;318(7190):1023–24.

Creating a Conscious Kitchen

1. Ludwig DS, Ebbeling CB. The carbohydrate-insulin model of obesity: Beyond "calories in, calories out." *JAMA Intern Med.* 2018 Aug 1;178(8):1098–1103.

2. US Department of Agriculture National Agriculture Library. Organic Aquaculture. https://www.nal.usda.gov/afsic/organic-aquaculture. June 2016.

3.   Worthington V. Nutritional quality of organic versus conventional fruits, vegetables, and grains. *J Altern Complement Med.* 2001 Apr;7(2):161–73.

4.   Priyadarshi A, Khuder SA, Schaub EA, et al. A meta-analysis of Parkinson's disease and exposure to pesticides. *Neurotoxicology.* 2000 Aug; 21(4)435–40.

5.   Uribarri J, Woodruff S, Goodman S, et al. Advanced Glycation end products in foods and a practical guide to their reduction in the diet. *J Am Diet Assoc.* 2010;110(6):911–16.e12. doi:10.1016/j.jada.2010.03.018.

RECIPE INDEX

NUTRITIONAL ANALYSIS INDEX

RECIPE	NUTRITIONAL ANALYSIS
African Sweet Potato Stew from Hugh Jackman	Per Serving: Calories: 313, Fat: 21 g, Saturated Fat: 3 g, Cholesterol: 0 mg, Fiber: 9 g, Protein: 9 g, Carbohydrates: 26 g, Sodium: 897 mg
Almond Cauliflower Fritters	Per Fritter: Calories: 41, Fat: 3 g, Saturated Fat: 0 g, Cholesterol: 0 mg, Fiber: 1 g, Protein: 2 g, Carbohydrates: 3 g, Sodium: 130 mg
Almond Chicken Skewers with Green Beans	Per Serving: Calories: 509, Fat: 28 g, Saturated Fat: 4 g, Cholesterol: 102 mg, Fiber: 8 g, Protein: 49 g, Carbohydrates: 21 g, Sodium: 754 mg
Anti-Aging Asparagus Soup	Per Serving: Calories: 262, Fat: 17 g, Saturated Fat: 3 g, Cholesterol: 0 mg, Fiber: 5 g, Protein: 8 g, Carbohydrates: 25 g, Sodium: 1200 mg
Avocado Mayo	Per 2 Tablespoon Serving: Calories: 251, Fat: 28 g, Saturated Fat: 3 g, Cholesterol: 30 mg, Fiber: 0 g, Protein: 1 g, Carbohydrates: 0 g, Sodium: 206 mg
Bison Wraps with Poblano-Avocado Sauce	Per Serving: Calories: 574, Fat: 36 g, Saturated Fat: 5 g, Cholesterol: 121 mg, Fiber: 6 g, Protein: 41 g, Carbohydrates: 24 g, Sodium: 2623 mg
Blushing Beet Dip	Per 2 Tablespoon Serving: Calories: 151, Fat: 13 g, Saturated Fat: 2 g, Cholesterol: 0 mg, Fiber: 3 g, Protein: 4 g, Carbohydrates: 7 g, Sodium: 473 mg
Broccoli Breakfast Bowl	Per Serving: Calories: 460, Fat: 33 g, Saturated Fat: 6 g, Cholesterol: 373 mg, Fiber: 9 g, Protein: 26 g, Carbohydrates: 22 g, Sodium: 542 mg
Buckwheat Blini with Smoked Salmon and Spinach	Per Serving: Calories: 435, Fat: 15 g, Saturated Fat: 5 g, Cholesterol: 88 mg, Fiber: 8 g, Protein: 43 g, Carbohydrates: 38 g, Sodium: 625 mg

Butternut Taco Wraps with Hemp Seed Cream

Per Serving: Calories: 295, Fat: 16 g, Saturated Fat: 2 g, Cholesterol: 0 mg, Fiber: 10 g, Protein: 10 g, Carbohydrates: 32 g, Sodium: 1398 mg

Cacao–Brazil Nut Bites

Per Serving: Calories: 110, Fat: 9 g, Saturated Fat: 4 g, Cholesterol: 0 mg, Fiber: 2 g, Protein: 2 g, Carbohydrates: 8 g, Sodium: 75 mg, Sugars: 5 g

Cacao-Coconut Custard

Per Serving: Calories: 322, Fat: 19 g, Saturated Fat: 14 g, Cholesterol: 0 mg, Fiber: 8 g, Protein: 5 g, Carbohydrates: 32 g, Sodium: 70 mg, Sugars: 22 g

Cajun Spice Blend

Per 2 Tablespoon Serving: Calories: 35, Fat: 1 g, Saturated Fat: 0 g, Cholesterol: 0 mg, Fiber: 3 g, Protein: 2 g, Carbohydrates: 8 g, Sodium: 1378 mg

Carrot Ginger Dressing

Per 2 Tablespoon Serving: Calories: 52, Fat: 5 g, Saturated Fat: 1 g, Cholesterol 0 mg, Fiber: 0 g, Protein: 0 g, Carbohydrates: 1 g, Sodium: 65 mg

Chermoula Cauliflower Steaks

Per Serving: Calories: 717, Fat: 61 g, Saturated Fat: 8 g, Cholesterol: 0 mg, Fiber: 15 g, Protein: 17 g, Carbohydrates: 39 g, Sodium: 1482 mg

Chicken and Apple Salad

Per Serving: Calories: 704, Fat: 48 g, Saturated Fat: 7 g, Cholesterol: 130 mg, Fiber: 5 g, Protein: 44 g, Carbohydrates: 24 g, Sodium: 2065 mg, Sugars: 15 g

Chicken Bone Broth from Chef Marco Canora

Per 1 Cup Serving: Calories: 585, Fat: 52 g, Saturated Fat: 0 g, Cholesterol: 167 mg, Fiber: 1 g, Protein: 27 g, Carbohydrates: 4 g, Sodium: 271 mg

Chocolate-Almond Sandwich Cookies

Per Serving (does not include optional maple syrup): Calories: 447, Fat: 38 g, Saturated Fat: 16 g, Cholesterol: 62 mg, Fiber: 4 g, Protein: 7 g, Carbohydrates: 24 g, Sodium: 254 mg, Sugars: 11 g

Chocolate Caramel Almond-Butter Cups

Per Cup: Calories: 236, Fat: 19 g, Saturated Fat: 13 g, Cholesterol: 0 mg, Fiber: 1 g, Protein: 2 g, Carbohydrates: 16 g, Sodium: 51 mg, Sugars: 13 g

Clean Ketchup

Per 2 Tablespoon Serving: Calories: 41, Fat: 0 g, Saturated Fat: 0 g, Cholesterol: 0 mg, Fiber: 3 g, Protein: 2 g, Carbohydrates: 8 g, Sodium: 405 mg

Coconut Chutney **from Mark Bittman**	Per 2 Tablespoon Serving: Calories: 37, Fat: 3 g, Saturated Fat: 3 g, Cholesterol: 0 mg, Fiber: 1 g, Protein: 1 g, Carbohydrates: 2 g, Sodium: 21 mg
Coconut-Pecan Yam Bake **from Dr. Deanna Minich**	Per Serving (does not include honey): Calories: 180, Fat: 10 g, Saturated Fat: 5 g, Cholesterol: 0 g, Fiber: 5 g, Protein: 3 g, Carbohydrates: 23 g, Sodium: 56 mg
Coriander Salmon with **Coconut-Tomato Salsa**	Per Serving: Calories: 453, Fat: 30 g, Saturated Fat: 13 g, Cholesterol: 105 mg, Fiber: 5 g, Protein: 33 g, Carbohydrates: 14 g, Sodium: 1283 mg
Crazy Sexy Trail Mix **from Kris Carr**	Per 2 Tablespoon Serving: Calories: 159, Fat: 13 g, Saturated Fat: 3 g, Cholesterol: 0 mg, Fiber: 2 g, Protein: 4 g, Carbohydrates: 10 g, Sodium: 8 mg, Sugars: 5 g
Creamy Truffle Spaghetti **Squash with Tempeh**	Per Serving: Calories: 887, Fat: 75 g, Saturated Fat: 12 g, Cholesterol: 0 mg, Fiber: 12 g, Protein: 30 g, Carbohydrates: 36 g, Sodium: 1814 mg
Crispy Carrot Fries **with Pesto**	Per Serving: Calories: 466, Fat: 41 g, Saturated Fat: 6 g, Cholesterol: 0 mg, Fiber: 7 g, Protein: 6 g, Carbohydrates: 23 g, Sodium: 832 mg
Dairy-Free Queso	Per 2 Tablespoon Serving: Calories: 75, Fat: 6 g, Saturated Fat: 1 g, Cholesterol: 0 mg, Fiber: 2 g, Protein: 3 g, Carbohydrates: 4 g, Sodium: 201 mg
Delicata Buckwheat Bowls	Per Serving: Calories: 308, Fat: 15 g, Saturated Fat: 5 g, Cholesterol: 0 mg, Fiber: 11 g, Protein: 11 g, Carbohydrates: 40 g, Sodium: 907 mg
Easy Homemade **Teriyaki Sauce**	Per 2 Tablespoon Serving: Calories: 41, Fat: 1 g, Saturated Fat: 0 g, Cholesterol: 0 mg, Fiber: 0 g, Protein: 3 g, Carbohydrates: 6 g, Sodium: 1406 mg
Easy Sesame Super Greens	Per Serving: Calories: 143, Fat: 11 g, Saturated Fat: 1 g, Cholesterol: 0 mg, Fiber: 4 g, Protein: 6 g, Carbohydrates: 10 g, Sodium: 543 mg
Eggplant Moussaka	Per Serving: Calories: 684, Fat: 52 g, Saturated Fat: 21 g, Cholesterol: 139 mg, Fiber: 11 g, Protein: 28 g, Carbohydrates: 30 g, Sodium: 611 mg

Eggs and Peppers from Dr. Mehmet Oz	Per Serving: Calories: 490, Fat: 35 g, Saturated Fat: 16 g, Cholesterol: 373 mg, Fiber: 8 g, Protein: 17 g, Carbohydrate: 31 g, Sodium: 152 mg
Everything Vinaigrette	Per 2 Tablespoon Serving: Calories: 234, Fat: 25 g, Saturated Fat: 3 g, Cholesterol: 0 mg, Fiber: 1 g, Protein: 1 g, Carbohydrates: 3 g, Sodium: 194 mg
Farmers' Market Muffins	Per Serving (does not include maple syrup): Calories: 271, Fat: 21 g, Saturated Fat: 2 g, Cholesterol: 56 mg, Fiber: 4 g, Protein: 8 g, Carbohydrates: 16 g, Sodium: 189 mg, Sugars: 10 g
Favorite Hummus from Gisele Bündchen and Tom Brady	Per 2 Tablespoon Serving: Calories: 84, Fat: 6 g, Saturated Fat: 1 g, Cholesterol: 0 mg, Fiber: 2 g, Protein: 3 g, Carbohydrates: 6 g, Sodium: 79 mg
Feel-Good Pesto Steak Salad	Per Serving: Calories: 1002, Fat: 76 g, Saturated Fat: 11 g, Cholesterol: 109 mg, Fiber: 13 g, Protein: 58 g, Carbohydrates: 33 g, Sodium: 679 mg
Flourless Protein Power Bread	Per Serving: Calories: 632, Fat: 57 g, Saturated Fat: 7 g, Cholesterol: 140 mg, Fiber: 11 g, Protein: 22 g, Carbohydrates: 17 g, Sodium: 495 mg
Forbidden Rice No-Fry Stir-Fry	Per Serving: Calories: 393, Fat: 18 g, Saturated Fat: 2 g, Cholesterol: 0 mg, Fiber: 14 g, Protein: 16 g, Carbohydrates: 48 g, Sodium: 1099 mg
Golden Cauliflower Caesar Salad	Per Serving: Calories: 368, Fat: 33 g, Saturated Fat: 5 g, Cholesterol: 0 mg, Fiber: 7 g, Protein: 8 g, Carbohydrates: 16 g, Sodium: 964 mg
Go-To Cremini Chili	Per Serving: Calories: 556, Fat: 31 g, Saturated Fat: 12 g, Cholesterol: 116 mg, Fiber: 11 g, Protein: 36 g, Carbohydrates: 37 g, Sodium: 624 mg
Grab-and-Go Jerky	Per 2 Ounce Serving: Calories: 197, Fat: 5 g, Saturated Fat: 2 g, Cholesterol: 87 mg, Fiber: 0 g, Protein: 36 g, Carbohydrates: 2 g, Sodium: 1389 mg
Grain-Free Cauliflower Tabbouleh	Per Serving: Calories: 205, Fat: 14 g, Saturated Fat: 2 g, Cholesterol: 0 mg, Fiber: 5 g, Protein: 5 g, Carbohydrates: 17 g, Sodium: 485 mg

Grain-Free Lemon-Blueberry Pancakes	Per Serving (does not include honey or maple syrup): Calories: 127, Fat: 7 g, Saturated Fat: 4 g, Cholesterol: 93 mg, Fiber: 2 g, Protein: 4 g, Carbohydrates: 12 g, Sodium: 83 mg, Sugars: 3 g
Grass-Fed Ghee	Per 2 Tablespoon Serving: Calories: 199, Fat: 23 g, Saturated Fat: 14 g, Cholesterol: 57 mg, Fiber: 0 g, Protein: 0 g, Carbohydrates: 0 g, Sodium: 0 mg
Grass-Fed Sliders on Sweet Potato UnBuns from Dave Asprey	Per One Slider: Calories: 322, Fat: 18 g, Saturated Fat: 4 g, Cholesterol: 84 mg, Fiber: 7 g, Protein: 14 g, Carbohydrates: 28 g, Sodium: 469 mg
Greek Spice Rub	Per 2 Tablespoon Serving: Calories: 28, Fat: 0 g, Saturated Fat: 0 g, Cholesterol: 0 mg, Fiber: 2 g, Protein: 1 g, Carbohydrates: 6 g, Sodium: 1176 mg
Green Goodness Dressing	Per 2 Tablespoon Serving: Calories: 104, Fat: 11 g, Saturated Fat: 2 g, Cholesterol: 0 mg, Fiber: 1 g, Carbohydrates: 2 g, Sodium: 169 mg
Green Shakshuka	Per Serving: Calories: 241, Fat: 19 g, Saturated Fat: 14 g, Cholesterol: 187 mg, Fiber: 1 g, Protein: 8 g, Carbohydrates: 8 g, Sodium: 378 mg
Hemp Seed Bread from Cam Sims	Per Serving: Calories: 324, Fat: 21 g, Saturated Fat: 2 g, Cholesterol: 0 mg, Fiber: 11 g, Protein: 15 g, Carbohydrates: 27 g, Sodium: 300 mg, Sugars: 6 g
Herb and Beet Boston Salad	Per Serving: Calories: 513, Fat: 35 g, Saturated Fat: 5 g, Cholesterol: 0 mg, Fiber: 15 g, Protein: 15 g, Carbohydrates: 42 g, Sodium: 1073 mg
Herbed Mini Meatballs with Butternut Noodles	Per Serving: Calories: 488, Fat: 30 g, Saturated Fat: 7 g, Cholesterol: 169 mg, Fiber: 8 g, Protein: 33 g, Carbohydrates: 26 g, Sodium: 736 mg
Herbed Sardine Cakes with Avocado-Broccoli Salad	Per Serving (does not include honey): Calories: 603, Fat: 46 g, Saturated Fat: 7 g, Cholesterol: 137 mg, Fiber: 12 g, Protein: 30 g, Carbohydrates: 26 g, Sodium: 1061 mg
Immune-Boosting Bone Broth	Per 1 Cup Serving: Calories: 1064, Fat: 69 g, Saturated Fat: 27 g, Cholesterol: 330 mg, Fiber: 4 g, Protein: 90 g, Carbohydrates: 17 g, Sodium: 1128 mg

Kale, Carrot, and Avo Salad with Tahini Dressing from Gwyneth Paltrow

Per Serving: Calories: 504, Fat: 37 g, Saturated Fat: 5 g, Cholesterol: 0 mg, Fiber: 18 g, Protein: 17 g, Carbohydrates: 37 g, Sodium: 228 mg

---

Lamb Skewers with Roasted Carrots

Per Serving: Calories: 803, Fat: 62 g, Saturated Fat: 16 g, Cholesterol: 130 mg, Fiber: 7 g, Protein: 39 g, Carbohydrates: 24 g, Sodium: 1364 mg

---

Lemon-Berry Rose Cream Cake

Per Serving: Calories: 397, Fat: 30 g, Saturated Fat: 10 g, Cholesterol: 0 mg, Fiber: 4 g, Protein: 9 g, Carbohydrates: 28 g, Sodium: 18 mg, Sugars: 16 g

---

Lemon–Poppy Seed Shortbread Bites

Per Serving: Calories: 119, Fat: 11 g, Saturated Fat: 8 g, Cholesterol: 0 mg, Fiber: 2 g, Protein: 3 g, Carbohydrates: 4 g, Sodium: 14 mg

---

Maple Harvest Crisp

Per Serving: Calories: 388, Fat: 30 g, Saturated Fat: 7 g, Cholesterol: 0 mg, Fiber: 8 g, Protein: 9 g, Carbohydrates: 28 g, Sodium: 77 mg, Sugars: 18 g

---

Maple Pumpkin Pie from Danielle Walker

Per Serving: Calories: 402, Fat: 25 g, Saturated Fat: 9 g, Cholesterol: 111 mg, Fiber: 5 g, Protein: 10 g, Carbohydrates: 37 g, Sodium: 187 mg, Sugars: 18 g

---

Medicinal Mushroom Tonic

Per Serving (does not include maple syrup): Calories: 119, Fat: 12 g, Saturated Fat: 11 g, Cholesterol: 0 mg, Fiber: 1 g, Protein: 1 g, Carbohydrates: 4 g, Sodium: 2 mg

---

Mediterranean Lentil Stew

Per Serving: Calories: 225, Fat: 6 g, Saturated Fat: 1 g, Cholesterol: 0 mg, Fiber: 8 g, Protein: 11 g, Carbohydrates: 35 g, Sodium: 1421 mg

---

Mediterranean Trout en Papillote

Per Serving: Calories: 299, Fat: 15 g, Saturated Fat: 3 g, Cholesterol: 75 mg, Fiber: 3 g, Protein: 28 g, Carbohydrates: 12 g, Sodium: 178 mg

---

Mexican Chicken Salad

Per Serving: Calories: 540, Fat: 34 g, Saturated Fat: 5 g, Cholesterol: 88 mg, Fiber: 8 g, Protein: 37 g, Carbohydrates: 25 g, Sodium: 1069 mg

---

Middle Eastern Lamb Liver with Parsley Salad from Dr. Terry Wahls

Per Serving: Calories: 401, Fat: 24 g, Saturated Fat: 8 g, Cholesterol: 576 mg, Fiber: 2 g, Protein: 36 g, Carbohydrates: 9 g, Sodium: 139 mg

---

Millet Porridge with Roasted Stone Fruit	Per Serving (does not include maple syrup): Calories: 403, Fat: 27 g, Saturated Fat: 18 g, Cholesterol: 0 mg, Fiber: 8 g, Protein: 12 g, Carbohydrates: 33 g, Sodium: 106 mg, Sugars: 8 g
Morning Glory Collagen Smoothie	Per Serving: Calories: 317, Fat: 18 g, Saturated Fat: 6 g, Cholesterol: 0 mg, Fiber: 7 g, Protein: 26 g, Carbohydrates: 18 g, Sodium: 178 mg
Moroccan Fish Balls in Pepper Sauce	Per Serving: Calories: 430, Fat: 27 g, Saturated Fat: 4 g, Cholesterol: 83 mg, Fiber: 7 g, Protein: 18 g, Carbohydrates: 32 g, Sodium: 1355 mg
Mussels and Fennel in White Wine	Per Serving: Calories: 335, Fat: 14 g, Saturated Fat: 4 g, Cholesterol: 46 mg, Fiber: 5 g, Protein: 18 g, Carbohydrates: 23 g, Sodium: 664 mg
No-Bake Carrot Mini Cupcakes	Per 1 Mini Cupcake: Calories: 228, Fat: 17 g, Saturated Fat: 8 g, Cholesterol: 0 mg, Fiber: 3 g, Protein: 3 g, Carbohydrates: 20 g, Sodium: 60 mg, Sugars: 14 g
Orange-Blackberry Almond Scones	Per Serving (does not include coconut sugar): Calories: 337, Fat: 26 g, Saturated Fat: 6 g, Cholesterol 62 mg, Fiber: 6 g, Protein: 11 g, Carbohydrates: 19 g, Sodium: 204 mg
Out-of-This-World Alfredo	Per 2 Tablespoon Serving: Calories: 53, Fat: 4 g, Saturated Fat: 1 g, Cholesterol: 0 mg, Fiber 1 g, Protein: 2 g, Carbohydrates: 3 g, Sodium: 148 mg
Peppered Steaks with Roasted Oyster Mushrooms	Per Serving: Calories: 789, Fat: 77 g, Saturated Fat: 25 g, Cholesterol: 138 mg, Fiber: 4 g, Protein: 33 g, Carbohydrates: 13 g, Sodium: 1323 mg
Persian Green-Herb Omelet	Per Serving: Calories: 176, Fat: 12 g, Saturated Fat: 3 g, Cholesterol: 280 mg, Fiber: 2 g, Protein: 11 g, Carbohydrates: 7 g, Sodium: 698 mg
Poached-Egg Power Bowl	Per Serving: Calories: 320, Fat: 17 g, Saturated Fat: 4 g, Cholesterol: 373 mg, Fiber: 7 g, Protein: 18 g, Carbohydrates: 26 g, Sodium: 1070 mg, Sugars: 12 g
Pumpkin Cilantro Pesto	Per 2 Tablespoon Serving: Calories: 112, Fat: 10 g, Saturated Fat: 2 g, Cholesterol: 0 mg, Fiber: 1 g, Protein: 4 g, Carbohydrates: 2 g, Sodium: 157 mg

Raspberry Bliss Bars Per Bar: Calories: 149, Fat: 12 g, Saturated Fat: 5 g, Cholesterol: 0 mg, Fiber: 4 g, Protein: 4 g, Carbohydrates: 9 g, Sodium: 16 mg, Sugars: 3 g

Resistant-Starch Kitchari Per Serving: Calories: 354, Fat: 19 g, Saturated Fat: 11 g, Cholesterol: 0 mg, Fiber: 5 g, Protein: 8 g, Carbohydrates: 40 g, Sodium: 830 mg

Roasted Beet and Citrus Salad Per Serving: Calories: 420, Fat: 31 g, Saturated Fat: 4 g, Cholesterol: 0 mg, Fiber: 9 g, Protein: 8 g, Carbohydrates: 35 g, Sodium: 382 mg

Salted Pecan Fudge Cookies Per Cookie: Calories: 398, Fat: 35 g, Saturated Fat: 13 g, Cholesterol: 32 mg, Fiber: 5 g, Protein: 6 g, Carbohydrates: 19 g, Sodium: 305 mg, Sugars: 12 g

Savory Seed Crackers Per 8 Crackers: Calories: 277, Fat: 10 g, Saturated Fat: 1 g, Cholesterol: 0 mg, Fiber: 8 g, Protein: 10 g, Carbohydrates: 42 g, Sodium: 225 mg

Seared Scallops with Avocado-Yuzu Sauce Per Serving: Calories: 365, Fat: 31 g, Saturated Fat: 8 g, Cholesterol: 19 mg, Fiber: 5 g, Protein: 12 g, Carbohydrates: 14 g, Sodium: 1516 mg

Shepherd's Pie with Sweet Potato Topping from Dr. Drew Ramsey Per Serving: Calories: 372, Fat: 6 g, Saturated Fat: 5 g, Cholesterol: 59 mg, Fiber: 10 g, Protein: 23 g, Carbohydrates: 43 g, Sodium: 396 mg

Slow-Cooked Chicken Thighs with Kale Per Serving: Calories: 352, Fat: 11 g, Saturated Fat: 2 g, Cholesterol: 145 mg, Fiber: 6 g, Protein: 39 g, Carbohydrates: 23 g, Sodium: 934 mg

Slow-Cooked Lamb with Minty Millet Per Serving: Calories: 574, Fat: 35 g, Saturated Fat: 10 g, Cholesterol: 0 mg, Fiber: 6 g, Protein: 36 g, Carbohydrates: 31 g, Sodium: 384 mg

Slow-Roasted Salmon with Mustard Glaze from the Perlmutters Per Serving: Calories: 451, Fat: 32 g, Saturated Fat: 13 g, Cholesterol: 146 mg, Fiber: 1 g, Protein: 38 g, Carbohydrates: 2 g, Sodium: 179 mg

Smashed Persian Cucumbers Per Serving (does not include coconut sugar): Calories: 109, Fat: 10 g, Saturated Fat: 2 g, Cholesterol: 0 mg, Fiber: 2 g, Protein: 0 g, Carbohydrates: 7 g, Sodium: 683 mg

Smoked Fish Spread

Per 2 Tablespoon Serving: Calories: 82, Fat: 8 g, Saturated Fat: 1 g, Cholesterol: 13 mg, Fiber: 0 g, Protein: 3 g, Carbohydrates: 1 g, Sodium: 255 mg

Smoky Chipotle Ranch Dressing from Mark Sisson

Per 2 Tablespoon Serving: Calories: 127, Fat: 14 g, Saturated Fat: 3 g, Cholesterol: 16 mg, Fiber: 0 g, Protein: 0 g, Carbohydrates: 2 g, Sodium: 222 mg

Smoky Coconut Trail Mix

Per 2 Tablespoon Serving: Calories: 206, Fat: 18 g, Saturated Fat: 7 g, Cholesterol: 0 mg, Fiber: 3 g, Protein: 5 g, Carbohydrates: 8 g, Sodium: 150 mg, Sugars: 3 g

Soul Food Yam Soup

Per Serving: Calories: 303, Fat: 18 g, Saturated Fat: 2 g, Cholesterol: 0 mg, Fiber: 7 g, Protein: 8 g, Carbohydrates: 34 g, Sodium: 671 mg

Sparkling Emerald Tea

Per Serving: Calories: 10, Fat: 0 g, Saturated Fat: 0 g, Cholesterol: 0 mg, Fiber: 1 g, Protein: 0 g, Carbohydrates: 4 g, Sodium: 23 mg

Spiced Brazil Nut Milk

Per 1 Cup Serving: Calories: 443, Fat: 45 g, Saturated Fat: 11 g, Cholesterol: 0 mg, Fiber: 5 g, Protein: 10 g, Carbohydrates: 8 g, Sodium: 294 mg

Sticky Pomegranate Chicken Salad from Dr. Rupy Aujla

Per Serving (does not include pomegranate molasses): Calories: 845, Fat: 48 g, Saturated Fat: 6 g, Cholesterol: 55 mg, Fiber: 24 g, Protein: 42 g, Carbohydrates: 76 g, Sodium: 282 mg

Strawberry-Vanilla Chia Pudding

Per Serving (does not include honey): Calories: 601, Fat: 45 g, Saturated Fat: 28 g, Cholesterol: 0 mg, Fiber: 12 g, Protein: 17 g, Carbohydrates: 29 g, Sodium: 235 mg, Sugars: 14 g

Sunshine Seed Butter

Per 2 Tablespoon Serving: Calories: 235, Fat: 22 g, Saturated Fat: 6 g, Cholesterol: 0 mg, Fiber: 4 g, Protein: 6 g, Carbohydrates: 6 g, Sodium: 50 mg

Superfood Slaw

Per Serving: Calories: 504, Fat: 44 g, Saturated Fat: 6 g, Cholesterol: 0 mg, Fiber: 8 g, Protein: 8 g, Carbohydrates: 27 g, Sodium: 1125 mg, Sugars: 13 g

Superfood Smoothie Bowl

Per Serving: Calories: 601, Fat: 47 g, Saturated Fat: 17 g, Cholesterol: 0 mg, Fiber: 13 g, Protein: 14 g, Carbohydrates: 40 g, Sodium: 229 mg, Sugars: 19 g

Tahini Rainbow Cabbage Salad	Per Serving: Calories: 575, Fat: 47 g, Saturated Fat: 14 g, Cholesterol: 411 mg, Fiber: 7 g, Protein: 25 g, Carbohydrates: 19 g, Sodium: 1288 mg
Tangy Tomato Basil Sauce	Per 2 Tablespoon Serving: Calories: 20, Fat: 1 g, Saturated Fat: 0 g, Cholesterol: 0 mg, Fiber: 1 g, Protein: 1 g, Carbohydrates: 3 g, Sodium: 112 mg
Thai Broccoli Fish Stew	Per Serving: Calories: 487, Fat: 24 g, Saturated Fat: 15 g, Cholesterol: 70 mg, Fiber: 8 g, Protein: 35 g, Carbohydrates: 33 g, Sodium: 3259 mg
Tichi's Gazpacho from Chef José Andrés	Per Serving: Calories: 495, Fat: 43 g, Saturated Fat: 6 g, Cholesterol: 0 mg, Fiber: 6 g, Protein: 4 g, Carbohydrates: 24 g, Sodium: 1193 mg
Toasted-Caper and Salmon Salad	Per Serving: Calories: 460, Fat: 43 g, Saturated Fat: 6 g, Cholesterol: 10 mg, Fiber: 2 g, Protein: 12 g, Carbohydrates: 9 g, Sodium: 943 mg
Toasted Sage Butternut Pizza	Per Serving: Calories: 637, Fat: 48 g, Saturated Fat: 17 g, Cholesterol: 182 mg, Fiber: 11 g, Protein: 22 g, Carbohydrates: 32 g, Sodium: 1697 mg
Turkey Zucchini Lasagna	Per Serving: Calories: 577, Fat: 38 g, Saturated Fat: 12 g, Cholesterol: 155 mg, Fiber: 5 g, Protein: 41 g, Carbohydrates: 20 g, Sodium: 1830 mg
Turkish Halva	Per Piece: Calories: 140, Fat: 12 g, Saturated Fat: 2 g, Cholesterol: 0 mg, Fiber: 2 g, Protein: 4 g, Carbohydrates: 7 g, Sodium: 12 mg, Sugars: 4 g
Turmeric Collagen Elixir	Per Serving: Calories: 153, Fat: 0 g, Saturated Fat: 0 g, Cholesterol: 0 mg, Fiber: 1 g, Protein: 10 g, Carbohydrates: 19 g, Sodium: 41 mg
Turmeric Oil	Per 2 Tablespoon Serving: Calories: 244, Fat: 27 g, Saturated Fat: 3 g, Cholesterol: 0 mg, Fiber: 0 g, Protein: 0 g, Carbohydrates: 1 g, Sodium: 0 mg
Ultimate Mint Chocolate Shake	Per Serving (does not include dates): Calories: 279, Fat: 17 g, Saturated Fat: 2 g, Cholesterol: 0 mg, Fiber: 11 g, Protein: 20 g, Carbohydrates: 17 g, Sodium: 585 mg

Ultra-Creamy Cashew Butter Coffee	Per Serving: Calories: 214, Fat: 18 g, Saturated Fat: 5 g, Cholesterol: 0 mg, Fiber: 2 g, Protein: 6 g, Carbohydrates: 11 g, Sodium: 159 mg
Uplifting Herbal Hemp Latte	Per Serving: Calories: 274, Fat: 19 g, Saturated Fat: 6 g, Cholesterol: 0 mg, Fiber: 3 g, Protein: 10 g, Carbohydrates: 21 g, Sodium: 147 mg, Sugars: 16 g
Wild Rice–Stuffed Chicken	Per Serving: Calories: 661, Fat: 37 g, Saturated Fat: 9 g, Cholesterol: 104 mg, Fiber: 7 g, Protein: 35 g, Carbohydrates: 48 g, Sodium: 2074 mg
Wild Salmon Niçoise Salad	Per Serving: Calories: 608, Fat: 46 g, Saturated Fat: 7 g, Cholesterol: 247 mg, Fiber: 4 g, Protein: 35 g, Carbohydrates: 14 g, Sodium: 1166 mg
Zesty Mexican Seasoning	Per 2 Tablespoon Serving: Calories: 42, Fat: 1 g, Saturated Fat: 0 g, Cholesterol: 0 mg, Fiber: 3 g, Protein: 2 g, Carbohydrates: 8 g, Sodium: 1027 mg
Zesty Sautéed Summer Squash	Per Serving: Calories: 135, Fat: 11 g, Saturated Fat: 1 g, Cholesterol: 0 mg, Fiber: 2 g, Protein: 3 g, Carbohydrates: 9 g, Sodium: 302 mg
Zucchini Latkes with Lemon-Basil Guacamole	Per Serving: Calories: 542, Fat: 40 g, Saturated Fat: 8 g, Cholesterol: 187 mg, Fiber: 14 g, Protein: 23 g, Carbohydrates: 32 g, Sodium: 2560 mg

GENERAL INDEX

Paleo, 23–24
plant-based, 10, 36
USDA guidelines for, 18, 19, 30
vegan, 22–23, 24
See also Pegan Diet
dip, blushing beet, 148–49, 289
dopamine, 29
dressings
Caesar, 120–21
carrot ginger, 254–55, 290
green goodness, 266, 293
herb, 122
sesame, 153
smoky chipotle ranch, 274, 297
tahini, 123, 129, 294, 298
See also vinaigrette

E
edamame, stir-fry with, 212
eggplant, moussaka with, 194–95, 291
eggs
avocado mayo with, 250
breakfast bowl with, 70
cabbage salad with, 129
pancakes with, 75, 94
pasture-raised, 30–31, 46, 50
peppers and, 71, 292
Persian omelet with, 82–83
power bowl with, 84–85, 295
protein power bread with, 262–63
pumpkin pie filling with, 230
salmon Niçoise salad with, 132–33
shakshuka with, 76–77
Environmental Working Group (EWG), 44, 46, 47, 281, 282

F
Fair Trade Federation, 47, 281
farmers' markets, 6, 7
fats, 50
cooking with, 57, 58, 60–61
healthy, 32, 35
in Paleo diet, 24
saturated, 19, 32
trans, 27, 32, 34
See also butter; oils
fatty acids
conjugated linoleic, 103
oleic, 250
omega-6, 47
pinolenic, 121
See also omega-3 fatty acids
FDA (Food and Drug Administration), 32
fennel, mussels and, 186–87, 295
fiber, 23, 24, 25, 34
fish, 49, 281
jerky made from, 49
Mediterranean trout, 182–83, 294
Moroccan cod balls, 184–85, 295
in Paleo diet, 23, 24
SMASH, 30, 32, 50
wild-caught or farmed, 30, 32, 46–47
See also salmon; sardines
flavonoids, 54
flaxseed
hemp seed bread with, 268–69
raspberry bars with, 106
foods
addiction to, 29, 43
additives in, 25, 27
choosing right, 43–55
connection through, 6, 12
consumer demand for quality, 10–11

cost and access to, 7–8
government policies for, 8, 17–20
grass-fed or pasture-raised, 46, 281
health and, 11–12, 16, 18–19, 27
labeling of, 10–11, 17, 19, 27, 43–47
local, 6–7, 282
marketing of, 5, 7, 12, 19, 43, 44, 47
pantry staple, 49–55
personal philosophy of, 10, 16–17
research on, 8
resources for, 281–83
food stamp program, 18
fritters, almond cauliflower, 98–99, 289
fruits, 50
colorful, 54–55
government subsidies for, 18
low-glycemic, 29, 35
in Paleo diet, 23, 24

G
GAO (Government Accountability Office), 18
garlic
Alfredo sauce with, 267
asparagus soup with, 139
summer squash with, 160–61
sweet potato stew with, 136
gazpacho, Tichi's, 143, 298
ghee, 28
cooking with, 57, 60–61
grass-fed, 264–65, 293
ginger, 52
dressing with, 254–55, 290
smoothie bowl with, 91
sweet potato stew with, 136

gluten, 27–28
  aliases for, 43
  grains without, 28–29, 35
  resource for, 281
glyphosate, 27
GMOs (genetically modified
    organisms)
  avoiding, 27, 46, 282
  labeling of, 10–11, 17
goji berries, trail mix with,
    100
grains
  cereal, 19, 27
  gluten-free, 28–29, 35
  gluten in, 27–28
  soaking, 58
  whole, 49
grocery shopping, online,
    283
guacamole, lemon-basil,
    94–95, 299

H
halva, Turkish, 234–35,
    298
hazelnuts, pomegranate
    chicken salad with, 125
hemp oil, 70
hemp seeds
  bread with, 268–69, 293
  cream sauce with, 206–7,
    290
  latte with, 239, 299
  smoothie with, 79
herbs, 35
  dressing with, 122, 293
  medicinal, 50–52
  Persian omelet with,
    82–83, 295
  See also specific herb
honey
  buttercream frosting
    with, 233
  in Paleo diet, 23, 24
  in vegan diet, 22
hummus, 50
  favorite, 102, 292

Hyman, Mark, 4–7
  food philosophy of, 10,
    16–17
  Food: What the Heck
    Should I Eat?, 8, 23, 283
  resources of, 283

J
Jackman, Hugh, 136, 283,
    289
jerky, 49
  grab-and-go, 103, 292

K
kale
  chicken with, 169, 296
  Mediterranean stew with,
    137
  salad with, 123, 294
  shakshuka with, 76–77
ketchup, 25
  clean, 50, 256, 290
kimchi, 50
Kiss the Ground (Tickell), 30,
    281
kitchari, resistant starch,
    214–15, 296
kitchen tools, 63
knives, 63

L
lactose intolerance, 28
lamb, 46
  liver of, 198, 294
  skewers of, 197, 294
  slow-cooked, 202–3,
    296
lasagna, turkey zucchini,
    170–71, 298
latkes, 6
  zucchini, 94–95, 299
latte, herbal hemp, 239,
    299
leeks
  asparagus soup with, 139
  shakshuka with, 76–77
legumes, 34, 49, 58

lemon
  cake filling with, 226–27,
    294
  guacamole with, 94–95,
    299
  pancakes with, 74–75, 293
  pesto with, 155
  salads with, 117, 130
  shortbread bites with,
    104, 294
lentils, 34
  Mediterranean stew with,
    137, 294
  pomegranate chicken
    salad with, 125
  shepherd's pie with, 199
lettuce
  cauliflower Caesar salad
    with, 120–21
  herb and beet salad with,
    122
  tacos wrapped in, 206–7
  See also arugula
lifestyle diseases, 11–12
lime, Thai broccoli fish stew
    with, 144
lutein, 55, 250
lycopene, 55

M
macronutrients, 42
maple syrup
  fruit crisp with, 228–29,
    294
  pumpkin pie with, 230–31,
    294
marinades, 58
Marine Stewardship
    Council, 47, 281
mayonnaise, avocado, 50,
    250, 289
  recipes with, 109, 117, 274
MCT oil, 79, 91
meat
  cooking, 58
  grass-fed or pasture-
    raised, 30, 46, 50, 281

jerky made of, 49
in Paleo diet, 23, 24
villainization of, 22
See also beef; bison; lamb
Medicare and Medicaid, 18, 20
mercury, fish low in, 30, 32, 47
microbiome, 16
micronutrients, 42
milk, 28
dietary guidelines for, 19
spiced Brazil nut, 242–43, 297
See also almond milk; coconut milk
millet
lamb with minty, 202–3, 296
porridge of, 86–87, 295
scones with, 80–81
Minich, Deanna, 152, 283, 291
mint
chocolate shake with, 92–93, 298
dressings with, 118, 122
millet with, 202–3, 296
Moroccan fish balls with, 184
tea with, 240–41
turkey meatballs with, 168
miso, 50
moussaka, eggplant, 194–95, 291
Mozaffarian, Dariush, 18, 283
MSG (monosodium glutamate), 44
muffins, farmers' market, 101, 292
mung dal (split mung beans), kitchari with, 214–15
mushrooms
Alfredo sauce with, 267
chili with cremini, 140–41, 292

shepherd's pie with, 199
steaks with oyster, 200–201, 295
sweet potato stew with, 136
tonic of medicinal, 238, 294
mussels and fennel, 186–87, 295
mustard, 50
salmon glazed with, 188, 296

National Organic Program (NOP), 44, 283
Natural Resources Defense Council, 47, 281
Non-GMO Project, 46, 282
noodles, squash
Moroccan fish balls over, 185
turkey lasagna with, 170–71
turkey meatballs with, 168, 293
nuts, 49
cake crust with, 226
oils from, 57
protein power bread with, 262–63
soaking, 58
trail mixes with, 100, 110–11
See also almonds; Brazil nuts; cashews; hazelnuts; pecans; pine nuts; pistachios; walnuts

oats, 28–29
obesity, 8, 18–29, 42
oils, 49
black truffle, 208–9
hemp, 70
MCT, 79, 91
nut and seed, 57

sesame, 153, 291
turmeric, 276, 298
vegetable, 32, 34
See also avocado oil; coconut oil; olive oil
olive oil, 49
cooking with, 57
green goodness dressing with, 266
olives, salmon Niçoise salad with, 132–33
omega-3 fatty acids
foods high in, 32, 46, 88, 109, 133, 188, 207, 269, 273
vegan diet and, 22
omelet, Persian green-herb, 82–83, 295
onions
Mediterranean stew with, 137
pickled, 214
summer squash with, 160–61
orange
salad with beets and, 126–27, 296
scones with, 80–81, 295
oregano, 52, 137
organic foods, 44, 46, 282–83
Oz, Mehmet, 71, 283, 292

Paleo diet, 10, 23–24
Paltrow, Gwyneth, 123, 283, 294
pancakes
buckwheat blini, 72–73, 289
lemon-blueberry, 74–75, 293
zucchini latkes, 94–95, 299
pantry staples, 49
paprika, smoked, 111
parchment paper, baking fish in, 183

ABOUT THE AUTHOR

Mark Hyman, MD, believes that we all deserve a life of vitality—and that we have the potential to create it for ourselves. That's why he is dedicated to tackling the root causes of chronic disease by harnessing the power of functional medicine to transform health care. Dr. Hyman and his team work every day to empower people, organizations, and communities to heal their bodies and minds and to improve our social and economic resilience.

Dr. Hyman is a practicing family physician, an eleven-time *New York Times* best-selling author, and an internationally recognized leader, speaker, educator, and advocate in his field. He is the director of the

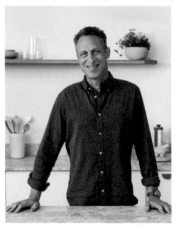

Cleveland Clinic Center for Functional Medicine. He is also the founder and medical director of The UltraWellness Center, chairman of the board of the Institute for Functional Medicine, a medical editor of *The Huffington Post*, and was a regular medical contributor on many television shows and networks, including *CBS This Morning, Today, Good Morning America,* CNN, *The View, Katie,* and *The Dr. Oz Show.*

Dr. Hyman works with individuals and organizations as well as policy makers and influencers. He has testified before both the White House Commission on Complementary and Alternative Medicine and the Senate Working Group on Health Care Reform on Functional Medicine. He has consulted with the surgeon general on diabetes prevention and participated in the 2009 White House Forum on Prevention and Wellness. Senator Tom Harkin of Iowa nominated Dr. Hyman for the President's Advisory Group on Prevention, Health Promotion, and Integrative and Public Health.

In addition, Dr. Hyman has worked with President Bill Clinton, presenting at the Clinton Foundation's Health Matters, Achieving Wellness in Every Generation conference and the Clinton Global Initiative, as well as with the World Economic Forum on global health issues. He is the winner of the Linus Pauling Award, the Nantucket Project Award, and the Christian Book of the Year Award for *The Daniel Plan,* and was inducted into the Books for Better Life Hall of Fame. Dr. Hyman also works with fellow leaders in his field to help people and communities thrive. Along with Rick Warren, Dr. Mehmet Oz, and Dr. Daniel Amen, he created the Daniel Plan, a faith-based initiative that helped the Saddleback Church collectively lose 250,000 pounds. He is an advisor and guest co-host on *The Dr. Oz Show,* and is on the board of Dr. Oz's HealthCorps, which tackles the obesity epidemic by educating American students about nutrition.

With Dr. Dean Ornish and Dr. Michael Roizen, Dr. Hyman crafted and helped introduce the Take Back Your Health Act of 2009 to the United States Senate to provide for reimbursement of lifestyle treatment of chronic disease. And with Tim Ryan in 2015, he helped introduce the ENRICH Act to Congress to fund nutrition in medical education. Dr. Hyman plays a substantial role in a major film produced by Laurie David and Katie Couric, released in 2014, called *Fed Up,* which addresses childhood obesity.

Please join him in helping us all take back our health at www.drhyman.com, or follow him on Twitter, Facebook, and Instagram.